The Everyperson's CPAP Handbook

2nd Edition

Elizabeth S. Lowe BGS, RPSGT, RST

i

DEDICATION

This book is dedicated to my mother Oralia, a woman of unparalleled wisdom and beauty who never lost faith in the person I could become; to my father Herbert, a man who loved us fiercely and was loved in return, may you rest with the angels and to my wonderful children, Charles, Johnathan and Jacqueline, my stalwart, my joy and my comfort.

PREFACE

The information in this book comes from years of hands-on interaction with patients, people who, like you, were looking for answers; seeking help, and trying to adjust to and incorporate the use of a CPAP machine into their daily routine.

It is, as the title states, a handbook, and should be utilized as such. It is meant to be used as a reference guide: a tool that will aid the newcomer and even the seasoned CPAP patient to address mask issues, machine maintenance, and ultimately guide the reader to satisfactory answers to their questions.

The first four chapters explain the mechanics of sleep apnea using analogies and stories derived from first-hand experience dealing with patients and their CPAP woes. While the topic of sleep apnea generally seems to be centered on the adult population, the mechanics of this disorder can affect from the youngest to the oldest. For those who have just been diagnosed, it will provide a greater understanding of the dangers posed by the sporadic nighttime breathing which is caused by apneas. For those suffering from constant sleepiness, or for those sleeping with someone who is restless, tossing and turning nightly, it may help them realize that the need for action is imperative

The subsequent chapters explain the types of masks, machines and secondary aids available to keep everything running smoothly. There are websites listed which will help you to find replacement parts, locate investigative aids that will make using CPAP more comfortable, or allow you to vent your frustrations or concerns on CPAP forums. In short, it is a book that helps the CPAP user get accustomed to using CPAP, minimizing the headaches involved in learning something new.

This book is not intended as a substitute for the medical advice of physicians. The reader should regularly consult a physician in matters relating to his/her health and particularly with respect to any symptoms that may require diagnosis or medical attention.

TABLE OF CONTENTS

CHAPTER ONE

Why am I so sleepy?

To sleep—perchance to dream: ay, there's the rub!

William Shakespeare – Hamlet

The first time I ever set foot into a sleep lab I was clueless about sleep. All I knew was that sleep entailed drifting into a sweet nothingness where time and conscious thought disappeared. I'd wake up with the sun shining through my window feeling rested and ready to start the day anew. It never occurred to me that, for many, when the sunset and the lights dimmed, a real-life horror story would unfold. Nightly, many people throughout the world suffer through hours of constant torture, being assaulted by the very thing that keeps us grounded to this planet. Gravity...

I remember sitting, that first night, watching the brainwaves of our four patients and wondering what they were thinking if they were even thinking, when suddenly the brainwaves of the first patient started to change. Within moments, the brainwaves of the other patients sequentially started to change in the same manner. I asked the tech what was happening and she replied. "Oh, they just went into REM." REM, rapid eye movement, or dreaming: It was the most fascinating thing I had ever seen. It was as if a sudden calm had overtaken the patients' minds. The brainwaves were small with waves that looked like miniature shark teeth scattered throughout the screen.

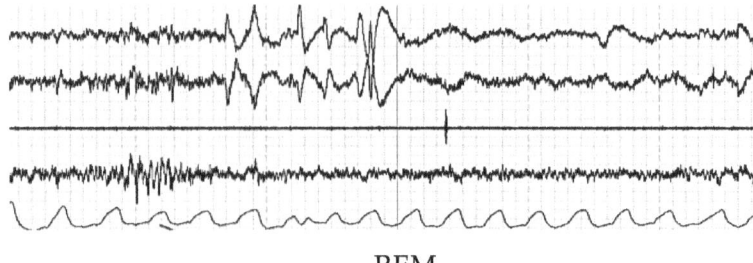

REM

Suddenly, the lines representing the eyes changed dramatically. Sharp peaks appeared, perfectly timed but flaring out in opposite directions. It looked like the outline of inkblots. I was hooked.

That night changed my life and set me on a path of discovery. I realized how beautiful sleep could be when it was graphically depicted on a computer screen and how blissful it was for the people sleeping, when they slept well. I learned that our brains are much more active at night than during the day and that the brain's main function was to prepare the body for the following day by guiding the body through several stages of sleep. Those stages were labeled stages 1, 2, and 3 or Slow Wave Sleep, (SWS for short), along with REM. To understand these stages, compare the act of falling asleep as walking into a cave. At the entrance, light and sound fills the mouth of the cave and we are aware of all that surrounds us. As we travel deeper into the cave, the bright light transitions to shades of gray erasing all detail. Our journey continues forward until we are blanketed in a sea of blackness and wrapped in a cocoon of silence.

Stage one sleep is similar to that transition between light and dark. We are somewhat aware of our surroundings, yet if awakened, we really can't remember any details. Stages 2 and 3 bring us down deeper into the cave of sleep. The outside world is non-existent to us as we rest in our ocean of calm. When we go into REM, our brain travels back up towards waking but not quite. This is the stage that most people consider our dream state and it is...though in actuality, we also dream in other stages of sleep.

It is here that we, in a sense, to go to the movies. The only difference is that in these movies we are active participants, stars in our own production, although they would not win us any academy awards. These personal movies are crazy and illogical, filled with objects and individuals we know as well as things that only our imagination or our sleeping minds can dream up.

Initially the REM stages are short and the non-REM stages are longer. Early on in the night, our bodies rest and recuperate. The brain takes care of the body by allowing it to repair and detoxify as we sleep. As we approach morning, our dream cycle gets longer. This allows our brain to take care of itself. I like to call dreaming the garbage disposal of the brain. It is at this time that we categorize all the necessary information and dream out the rest. Ideally, our brains cycle through these stages several times a night and once our brain has completed its job, and the body has rested sufficiently, we wake up; our bodies ready to take on a new day. In a perfect world, we would all sleep blissfully and wake up refreshed. But our world is not perfect.

All too often as I sat watching the monitors, I witnessed the suffering of those who were robbed of that gift of blissful sleep, most times unknowingly. I was presented with patients who were dragged in by their spouses, partners or other family members because they had witnessed odd breathing behavior that had scared them. The patients, on the other hand, were oblivious to this and were mainly in denial. I also noticed that any sleepiness was normally rationalized away by many of my patients. Common statements ranged from working erratic hours, to the children keeping them up, or the classic; having to get up to go to the bathroom several times a night. Some patients told me that they had been sleeping about 3-4 hours per night for years. Once, when my patient's wife complained about his difficulty sleeping at night, he responded. "I have no difficulty sleeping, I can fall asleep anywhere." And that is the problem in a nutshell. We are supposed to be AWAKE in the daytime and ASLEEP at night. If that is not happening that should be a warning sign that something is wrong.

No amount of coffee is going to fix the problem. I also see people who sleep with several pillows to help prop themselves up. Another common coping mechanism that I often hear about is the recliner. Many marriages have been "saved" by the spouses sleeping in separate bedrooms. Alcohol is another method my patients use to get to sleep. There is nothing wrong with having a beer or two before bed, or maybe a glass of wine to help the body unwind...right? Not at all! Not good. Alcohol, though thought to help the body fall asleep, actually does not allow the body to fall into that deep restorative sleep. It also may end up preventing the brain from entering the much needed REM state for as long as alcohol remains in the bloodstream. So, in short, using excuses to rationalize away that perpetual sleepiness normally doesn't work. It doesn't even buy us extra time. All it does is allow our symptoms to get worse. It surprises me how many people actually suffer from some form of sleeping disorder yet completely ignore their symptoms.

I was setting up an elderly Italian lady who had been accompanied by her daughters and niece to her sleep study because she could hardly speak English. She was a thin woman, not very tall, but she had been sent to have a sleep study because her family complained about her snoring. Two of the women had stayed in a hotel the previous night because they lived some distance away from the hospital. They were chatting with each other as I set up the patient and the conversation inevitably turned to the reason they were there. They were describing how the patient snored when one of the women turned to the cousin and said. "You were really snoring last night. I could hardly sleep!" They all laughed and they started recounting other instances when they had been subjected to having to suffer through sleepless nights listening to their cousin snoring. The cousin was a somewhat heavier than the other women. What struck me was that her neck was substantially thicker than average. I didn't make any comments as I continued setting up the patient. I wanted to ask if the snoring was rhythmic or erratic. Did they notice if she tossed and turned all night long, or if they had witnessed any jerking movements while she was sleeping, especially before she snored. Remember I mentioned gravity? Here is where it comes into play.

When we are awake and moving around gravity is pushing down from the top of our heads through to our feet. So gravity is not affecting our airway because it's flowing parallel to our windpipe or trachea. When it's time to go to sleep, we normally lie down. Now gravity is perpendicular to the trachea. When we fall asleep our muscles relax, including the muscles in the neck. There are many factors that can contribute to problems breathing at night including but not limited to excessive weight, enlarged tonsils, a thick tongue, a long uvula (the "bell" that is at the back of our throats) or a narrow airway. It can even be a combination of factors. Some of you may have heard the word "crowding" used by doctors to describe what exists in the throat. The point is that gravity is pushing down on our throats. It can be compared to bench pressing. Yes, bench pressing is mainly a guy thing, but even though sleep apnea primarily affects men, women and children cannot be counted out that easily.

Imagine yourself lying face up on the bench holding on to the bar. The more weight that is placed on the bar, the harder it is to push up against that weight. If too much weight is placed on the bar, the muscles give out, the bar falls on the neck and our windpipe is closed off. Fortunately, a trusty spotter at the gym can prevent this tragedy. Unfortunately, there is no one there to protect us when this happens at night. I have heard an innumerable number of times about the countless elbow jabs, or complaints delivered by my patients' respective spouses, partners, or significant others. I have also been told how frightening it is to the person watching when they see that no breathing is occurring. Patients have told me that others have counted the seconds as they ticked by, thinking that the event that they were witnessing could easily kill their partner. As the prolonged pauses in breathing crawled by, many stated that they wondered if the person with whom they were sharing their bed would drop dead right in front of them. But, believe me when I tell you that they only catch a small percentage of the times when this happens and unless we could move to a zero gravity environment like outer space, for example, where we could float around, gravity will always be our constant nemesis, ready to shut off our airway when we are asleep at night. OK, so if you are still asking yourself if it really is that bad, the answer is YES!!!

I often ask my patients to define sleep apnea. "It's when you stop breathing" is the most common response. But what happens when you stop breathing? First off, our brains expect us to breathe continuously throughout the entire night. So when we stop breathing, our brains are totally unprepared for this. So imagine that you are lying down breathing in and out and you have an event where you stop breathing. Because, your brain expects you to take in the next breath, it doesn't prepare the body to be without air. Hence, you have no reserves that your body can draw from. To understand this while you are awake and reading this, do the following…

STOP BREATHING NOW !!! Hold your breath for as long as you can. No cheating! No taking a deep breath beforehand. As you are reading this and holding your breath, you should start feeling minor anxiety because your brain is now realizing that the air supply has been shut down. Continue reading as your need to breathe starts to increase and your lungs want to expand to get the air in. If you are fit enough, you may still be holding your breath. Many of you have probably breathed in by now. Because you are sitting, awake and reading this, you CAN take that in breath and give your brain what it needs. But this happens when you are <u>sleeping!</u> That means that your airway has been blocked off and your brain can't get the air it needs. In a sense, you are being choked or you are actually suffocating every time you cannot breathe. This "choking" can last up to two minutes at times, depending on the severity of the person's sleep apnea. So what happens next?

The brain then protects itself and the vital organs by slowing down the flow of blood to the legs and arms. I have had patients tell me that many times they wake up with a tingly sensation in their extremities. One of the reasons could be sleep apnea. Why? Simply put, we can live without our extremities, but we cannot live without our heart, brain and other organs.

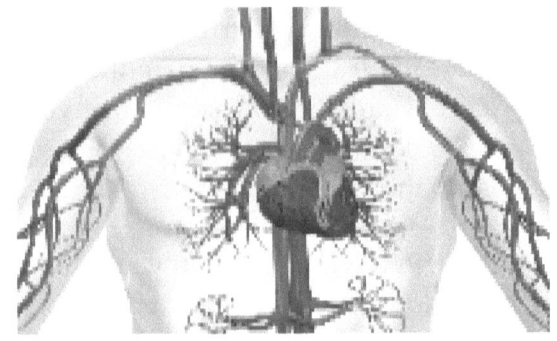

The previous illustration shows how the blood flows from the heart, through the body, starting from the largest arteries to the smallest capillaries and back again through the veins to the largest vein known as the Vena Cava back up to the heart.

The light grey in the picture is the blood that has very little oxygen, while the black represents the blood that is full of life giving oxygen. When the body has an event, the brain tries to get the air in through the nose because, in a perfect world, we all would breathe in and out through our noses while we slept. It's because our noses were designed to warm, moisten and filter the air before it enters the lungs. But because the trachea is blocked, no air can get in. The brain doesn't realize that immediately. It is only concerned with getting in the air. Since the nose isn't "working", the brain then decides to try and get in the air another way, namely, the mouth. So the jaw is dropped and again the brain tries to get the air in, obviously with no luck. By this time, the stress suffered by the body and brain is extreme.

Meanwhile, the heart keeps pumping, the liver and kidneys keep filtering, the cells keep producing energy and so on and so forth. As the oxygen level drops, the brain, which uses 20% of the oxygen we breathe in, is one of the first organs to be severely affected. The brain is now starving and brain cells begin to die. As the seconds tick by, the oxygen that is in the bloodstream continues to plummet. All the while, the brain continues to send the signal to get the air in by expanding the lungs and contracting the diaphragm. All this does is close the trachea even more. Remember trying to drink a thick milkshake with a straw? Remember how the straw would collapse when we sucked because the liquid would get stuck in the straw. Also recall that if we tried sucking harder it only caused the straw to flatten even more. That is exactly what happens to the trachea when you are having an "event" because we use the sucking motion to move air into our body as we breathe.

Finally, the brain realizes that there is something blocking the movement of air in and out of the body, so it sends out a stress hormone to jumpstart everything. Why a stress hormone? Well, remember that anxiety you were feeling when you were holding your breath earlier? That was stress, and it only lasted a few seconds,. At night, though, the time that can go by until the body can breathe again is normally a lot longer, so the body's stress level will be significantly more than any stress suffered while awake.

So the brain floods the body with **CORTISOL**. Cortisol is the stress hormone that acts as the on-off switch for the flight or fight reflex. That is when adrenaline is released into the body tensing the muscles including the ones in the throat and opening up the airway. Because the body is so deprived of air at this point, the air is inhaled more forcibly causing a very loud snore.

I recall a patient who I had when I worked as a night tech. I was watching him "sleeping" and having these events. On occasion, his body struggled for 90 seconds before it was able to open up the airway to get the air in. I watched as the oxygen level in his blood dropped to 54%. He would twitch and jerk during each event and when he was finally able to breathe, his snores were so loud, I could hear them through the walls of the lab. This particular patient had 189 events an hour. That meant that the instant he fell asleep, his airway would collapse. He was an extreme case and it took him years to get to that point, but it does show how well the body adapts to changes that occur to it over time. Obviously, he was perpetually tired and suffered from chronic sleep deprivation because he could fall asleep at the drop of a hat, but he was still working every day and getting through his daily obligations by drowning himself in coffee and taking naps at his desk when he had the time.

His lack of energy and mental grogginess were only part of his problem. Something much more serious was occurring. His sleep apnea was so severe that his body was actually flooded with cortisol 24 hours a day. What does that mean? Well cortisol, in small amounts, is good for the body. It helps to regulate many bodily functions and it is vital to our well-being. Unfortunately, too much cortisol triggers the body to store fat in the mid-section. It also causes fat to be stored in and around the vital organs. To further clarify what happens, imagine a steak marbled and ready for the grill. That marbling makes the meat tenderer because of the increased fat content. Great for eating but for our organs, that marbling contributes to the overall deterioration of our physical health.

It is no small wonder that my patient felt the way he did. He was obese with most of his weight centered on his waist, and he had also developed diabetes; possibly caused by too much cortisol in his system. I understand that most of you are thinking, "That isn't me", and I agree that 189 events an hour is extremely severe, but there are many who fall into the same category with far fewer events per hour.

I want to emphasize the importance of reducing the levels of cortisol in our systems by explaining its detrimental effects one other way; how it contributes to obesity. None of us actually can calculate how resilient our bodies are to the daily punishment we inflict upon them. Genetics plays a big part in determining the extent of our bodies' tolerance to what we do to them. I like comparing our bodies to cars. Some people can be compared to a high performance car like a Mercedes Benz or my favorite, an Audi, while other people are genetically more similar to an economy car like a Chevy or Hyundai. Both types of cars drive well when they are new. The engines purr, the suspension is tight and the interior is inviting. But, if the cars are not maintained by changing the oil regularly, rotating and balancing tires and checking the mechanics, etc. they will eventually start to break down. It is here that the difference between the qualities of the cars is most appreciated. The high performance cars will normally take much more abuse before succumbing to negative effects. The economy car will fail much more quickly.

For those people who have been blessed with genes that allow them to eat, drink and be merry and not feel the consequences immediately, consider yourself fortunate. For the genetically weaker of us, that type of lifestyle can wreak havoc to our systems. Even though our bodies tend to be very forgiving it is only a matter of time before things start to break down. This holds true for the comorbidities associated with sleep apnea. As this disorder nightly and methodically wears us down, our bodies slowly adjust to that change over the years while we are none the wiser. Our bodies respond to that negative force by developing high blood pressure, diabetes, and at times, congestive heart failure. At this point, if we were talking about a car, many people would just junk it and buy a new one; but unfortunately, we cannot change out our bodies for newer and improved models. We are stuck with the consequences brought on by our actions.

Can you imagine how different life would be if our bodies punished us by reacting negatively to anything that would cause it harm? CPAP would be non-existent and we would all be thin and full of vim and vigor. Obviously, this is not the case and here we are facing the biggest epidemic to face the human race. NO ONE WILL DENY THAT THEY LOVE TO EAT OR THAT THEY LOVE FOOD. We indulge in sweets; luscious morsels of decadent joy that stimulates our palates and release oodles of endorphins into our system. The fats we consume give our food a texture and smoothness augmenting the yum factor as we gingerly savor each bite or ravenously stuff our faces. I would never want to deprive anyone of his or her just dessert whether it is sweet, sour, salty or spicy. I would though, state the obvious.... Moderation is the key. Consider the animal kingdom. In nature, obesity does not exist. I look at some of my patients and wonder how they could have allowed their bodies to reach such large sizes. Could sleeping badly be the key?

I will reiterate…every time you stop breathing, your body goes into high alert. It sends out the cortisol to jump start the fight or flight reflex, which allows your adrenaline to flood your system and tighten your muscles including the muscles in your throat. The unfortunate side effect to that is that cortisol, in large quantities, tells the body to store fat in the midsection. The reason it tells the body to store the fat there is because it is suffering a lot of stress and normally when there is a stressful event that occurs, our bodies need energy fast! The body gets its energy from the liver and the liver makes energy from our stored fat. The area closest to our liver is our waist or more specifically our abdomen. Those lovely love handles, or that belly roll are supposed to serve a purpose. Unfortunately, in this day and age, they do not. We can blame our ancestors for this, because back when we were nomadic, roaming the land hunting and gathering, they were always in a state of alert. They truly lived by the axiom hunt or be hunted. They needed that quick energy boost when confronted with the local wildlife especially if it seemed that they were going to be the main course. Today, our stress levels are not nearly as severe, but unfortunately that biofeedback mechanism is still very active in our systems. To add insult to injury, when a body starts to store the fat it also produces an enzyme called **ghrelin**. The name of this hormone always reminds me of the movie Gremlins; and it wreaks as much havoc in our systems as those pesky creatures did in the movie. Excess fat causes more ghrelin to be produced by the body and the ghrelin makes the body scream FEED ME!!! It is an appetite stimulant.

Now if we were sleeping properly every night, no cortisol would be produced in excess, our bodies would regenerate and we would feel so much better in the morning. We may even begin to lose weight. With weight loss, the fat cells that have a direct line to the liver would reduce in size and that pesky ghrelin production would be greatly decreased. What would then happen is that our bodies would start producing more **leptin**. This hormone is an appetite suppressant. It tells the body that it should stop eating because it feels satiated or full.

So what does this mean in the world of CPAP? Well for those of you that have been diagnosed with sleep apnea who would love to find a way to get off the machine, it may be of benefit to you to lose the weight. Diet and exercise are, obviously, the old standards to achieve that goal as we have been told numerous times by endless experts; but to that, let me emphasize the importance of including your CPAP in the equation. It would be so self-defeating if all that work we do to improve our bodies should be negated by what happens to us at night.   If your goal is to lose weight, use that CPAP as a tool to reach that goal. I will repeat, it will stop the excess dumping of cortisol into your system and allow your body to slowly heal.   The inflammation that is occurring in your body will revert to a more normal state, blood pressure may start to stabilize and other maladies may be reversed or totally averted in time.

CHAPTER TWO

How bad can NOT breathing at night be for me?

"There is no stop; there is no interval between dreaming and waking. In this sense, it is possible to say: never, dreamer, can you awake"

Maurice Blanchot

There are degrees of sleep apnea. They are as follows: mild sleep apnea (5-15 events/hour), moderate sleep apnea (15-30 events/hour), and severe sleep apnea (30 events/hour and up). Yes, an individual who stops breathing a minimum of once every two minutes is considered severe...imagine that! So what does this mean? Well, a normal healthy adult can have 0-5 events/hour and live a perfectly normal life. Many doctors, though, start getting a bit nervous when a patient reaches 5 events per hour because of the increased stress that the body suffers through while the patient sleeps. Since the brain always try and protect itself and the vital organs, it will be constricting and expanding the arterioles to conserve the oxygen in the blood. That "slowing and speeding up" of the blood will eventually cause wear and tear on the body. It's similar to the wear and tear on the engine of a car. The constant stopping and starting that occurs with city driving, wears down the parts of an engine a lot faster, which is why mechanics say that if you have to buy a car with high mileage, it is preferable to buy one driven primarily on the highway. This is because highway driving puts less stress on the engine than city driving and if you are forced to buy a car with a lot of mileage, a car that racked up the miles on a highway will ultimately run more smoothly than a car driven around town.

Our circulatory system works in much the same way. If the rate of flow of the blood, or the blood pressure, has to be constantly regulated because we are not breathing properly through the night, over time the arteries will become inflamed. The inflammation will not only lead to high blood pressure; but with oxygen levels dipping constantly, the body may compensate by making more red blood cells. In this way, the body can store more oxygen. Good, right? Well… actually, no. What happens is that the body now has too many red blood cells. This makes the blood thick and sluggish. Now the heart has to pump harder to get the blood flowing around the body. So you are overexerting your heart in a bad way because your arteries are inflamed AND you have thick blood.

So nightly you sleep ignorant to everything that is happening to you. Continue on this downward spiral and you may end up developing a bevy of diseases including atherosclerosis. This happens when plaque starts building up on the sides of the walls of the arteries due to among other things, chronic inflammation. It is equivalent to developing hives on the inside of the body, but instead of the irregularities and lumpiness being caused from an allergic reaction they are caused by the chronic stress placed on the arterial walls. Recall how the skin appears when a person develops hives. The skin becomes inflamed in an irregular manner causing the skin to look and feel somewhat lumpy. Well that is what the inside of the artery wall looks like.

18

Plaque starts hitting the irregularities in the walls and eventually it will start to stick. The plaque builds up over time and hardens causing reduced blood flow and blockage. This blockage can lead to stroke and maybe even a heart attack. Yet, we blissfully go to sleep every night thinking that we will rest when instead; our body is dealing with exorbitantly high stress levels. For way too many of us this is a nightly occurrence. But it gets even better!

Imagine this; you are sleeping soundly when suddenly you stop breathing. The brain reacts by slowing everything down till it figures out what is wrong. As I said before, it eventually does and it signals the release of cortisol to start the fight or flight reflex in the body. This mechanism is used to flood the body with adrenaline. The muscles tighten up, the air rushes in and the body gets the oxygen it needs. It seems like the perfect solution. Unfortunately, all is not well in slumber land. When the lungs finally get the air and the oxygen is delivered to the bloodstream, the brain wants to get its share as quickly as possible. It accomplishes this by opening up the arteries so the blood can flow as quickly as possible. So now this wall of oxygen rich blood is barreling through the arteries at a proverbial breakneck speed.

You have the nice big arteries that flow into the medium sized arterioles down to the tiny, tiny capillaries. When the blood flow hits the capillaries, small ruptures start occurring. Do you recall the dramatic photos and video coverage of New Orleans in the aftermath of Hurricane Katrina? The levies in New Orleans did not break while there was no stress on the structure. They had been holding back the water for decades...but nothing like

19

Hurricane Katrina had slammed into the city: so as long as the waters of the Gulf remained calm, there was no need to worry. When Hurricane Katrina hit the coastline, it was the pounding on the weakened levies that caused the eventual breakdown and subsequent destruction to portions of said structures and the adjacent areas. Recall the vivid pictures and video footage of the water from the Gulf of Mexico passing through the breaks and spreading throughout the city inundating large areas and causing massive damage.

It is the same with the vessels in the body. Our capillaries are meant to accept red blood cells in single file in a nice orderly fashion. The reason that capillaries can only accept blood cells in single file is to allow enough time for the nutrients and waste to pass from the blood to the tissue and back. If there is a lot of blood rushing towards the capillaries, they will not be able to withstand the pressure placed upon them and breaks or ruptures of the capillaries will occur. These ruptures are termed small bleeds or ischemic strokes. It is then, through these ruptures, that the blood oozes out into the brain tissue causing irreparable and irreversible damage. This bleeding causes brain cells to die in frightening numbers. Granted, we may have a googol of brain cells but that does not mean that they are invaluable and are not needed.

Now imagine that an area is flooded, or there is roadwork, etc. that prevents us from getting from point A to point B in the most direct manner. We invariably search for an alternate route or a detour. It may take longer for us to get there but in the end we arrive at our destination.

Our nervous system works in a similar manner. Nerve cells are the only cells in the body that do not regenerate.

In other words, they don't heal themselves. So the nerves build an alternate route around the damaged area. But understand that even though the brain can "reroute" itself around the damaged parts and find a new pathway to do the same function, over time the lesions accumulate and the body can't compensate any longer. Compare this to driving in a city ridden with potholes. You can skirt the majority of them but eventually you will drive over one or several of them, which can ruin any vehicle over the course of time. So you try to avoid damaging your car and you slow down. You drive carefully around all the damaged areas on the roadway and eventually you arrive at your destination. Unfortunately, the trip has taken you significantly longer than you had originally anticipated. You are now agitated and frustrated. That is what happens in the brain. The nerve impulses that are sent have to be rerouted around the lesions caused by sleep apnea. So the impulses take longer to arrive. In short, your brain starts to slow down. Your memory starts to suffer. I call it being in a brain fog. Could it also be called dementia or perhaps a contributory factor in Alzheimer's?

There is ongoing clinical research to study if there is a correlation between sleep apnea and dementia. Irrespective of whether or not sleep apnea is a causal factor in dementia, let me give you some food for thought as you drift off to sleep. In the same way that lots of tiny fractures in the levies caused the massive break in New Orleans when Katrina hit; your brain can only withstand a certain amount of these small bleeds before a massive stroke occurs that we may or may not survive...so keep in mind...**Every time a person has an event, ischemic strokes can occur.**

Again, many of you may be thinking, "That isn't me" or "No one in my family has Alzheimer's or dementia". If that is the case then, good for you! So maybe you don't have dementia, but what is happening to your mental acuity? Do you find that your ability to bring up names, dates or certain words is getting more difficult? We all contribute this memory loss to our brains aging. Yet, new evidence has been discovered that shows that if we keep our brains active, our brains will remain sharp and we may be able to ward off dementia. So we all believe this and we play memory games, or puzzle games. We pick up a new hobby or learn to play a new instrument and we feel vindicated. We have helped our brains to get stronger and work faster; then the night descends and we lie down to sleep. Gravity then takes over and presses down on our throats. The airway is blocked and the oxygen starts to drop. All that effort and energy we have expended to keep our minds sharp during the day is negated by what happens to our bodies at night. We fall ever deeper in that downward spiral that starves our brains and hurts our bodies. The damage may not be as bad if your oxygen drops to the high 80's as opposed to the low 60"s, but starving your brain chronically will cause irreversible damage over time. You can only patch something up so many times before it breaks completely.

I saw an oxygen reading of 34% on a patient during an event when I was running a sleep study. Most doctors will agree that a reading as low as that from the pulse/oximeter would be considered artifact because they were not designed to accurately measure such low levels. To accurately measure the oxygen level when it drops that low a person has to undergo an arterial blood gas draw. It is normally done in a hospital setting and consists of drawing blood from the artery and measuring the blood oxygen level. But, if the oxygen level drops below 50% it is possible a person could suffer a heart attack. So, even if we don't succumb to a stroke; isn't it equally as horrifying to lose ourselves slowly in the murky grayness of a mind losing its ability to remember?

I think of my father. He was an extraordinarily handsome, strong man who took care of himself for most of his life. He never gained an ounce of weight and though he didn't exercise daily, especially as he got older, he kept himself entertained doing odd jobs around the house much to the dismay of my mother. I was visiting them one summer and I remember watching him while he was taking a nap. My mother and I were sitting on the adjoining sofa and I saw how his breathing paused. A few seconds went by. He didn't move an inch. He just lay there. Finally, he took in a deep breath and continued breathing. My father never snored, but the fact that I witnessed an event worried me. In retrospect, I think that he may have been suffering from central apneas where the brain "forgets" to breathe. I told my mother that he should be tested but she just brushed it off as nothing of major consequence and he never went for the study. He thought the same way. According to them, there could not be anything wrong, simply because he DIDN'T snore. A couple of years later, he suffered a major stroke. He became a shell of the man he once was and I wondered if things would have been different if he had heeded my advice. The funny thing was that he was terrified of having a stroke. This fear was further augmented when a friend of his suffered a stroke a few years earlier, but my father suffered from the same malady that most of us have: The idea that it could never happen to him. He thought that he was healthy. He thought that he did a good job of taking care of himself. He was wrong and there was nothing he could do when his brain failed him.

Genetics also plays a part in how our sleep patterns change over time. Some individuals are very sensitive to minor changes within themselves while some people are extremely resilient and can withstand decades of abuse before finally being brought into the lab by family members or other specialists. You can thank your family tree for that. Understand that we sleep away 30% of our lives. If our brain's main purpose is to prepare the body for the next day, then how important is it that it can do this efficiently?

I have already told you some of the negative effects of having severe sleep apnea. But what happens to people who have mild sleep apnea? Rest assured that even though the frequency of events may be greatly reduced, for all intents and purposes, the ultimate prognosis could be the same. Our brain can't perform the necessary functions to keep the body healthy because it is being constantly interrupted by the events that keep on blocking the airway. So our brain has to fix that problem before it can go back to its nightly functions. Soon the brain has developed a sleep debt. Depending on how long this continues and depending on the resilience of our bodies, that debt can affect our daily lives by causing us to be tired, lethargic and perpetually sleepy. Our daily dozing is caused by our brains trying to pay off some of that dept. When the events are frequent enough, the brain starts to prioritize. The need to get the job done can outweigh the need for oxygen; which is why oxygen levels can dip so dramatically. The brain is not a natural hoarder. It only wants what it needs to maintain homeostasis in the body. But it is almost forced to hoard because it cannot clear the body effectively while being interrupted by events. So it has to make a choice. It has to choose the lesser of two evils. Most of the time, when the apnea is sufficiently severe, it chooses to "clean house" over keeping the body oxygenated. The brain prefers to play Russian roulette with the body in order to get some of the vital processes needed to be accomplished completed before attending to opening the airway.

Our brains can only do so much while we sleep, as it struggles dealing with sleep apnea during the night. Sometimes the need to get the job done is so imperative that the brain will take whatever downtime you have available and send you off into slumber land. Pretty as that sounds, it is actually very dangerous because it can happen as we perform our daily routines. Think of the teacher who has to proctor an exam or the truck driver who has to take his load across the state or country. Think about the risks involved if an air traffic controller or a pilot who has untreated sleep apnea is allowed on the job. None of these people can allow sleep apnea to interfere with their job but it often does, and accidents can happen when they fall asleep. Only seconds need to pass for disasters to occur. In short, sleep apnea, regardless of the degree, puts undue stress and strain on the body.

To summarize, having sleep apnea may cause damage to the circulatory system, brain, plus diminish mental acuity and overall vim and vigor. Invariably, it's only a matter of time before the toll on the body becomes evident and at times irreversible all the while endangering the sufferer and those around him or her.

CHAPTER THREE

So what is a sleep study…and how many ways can I be monitored?

"You are the puppet and we are the puppeteers...but only for one night..."

Elizabeth Lowe

There are four accepted data collection methods now available when undergoing a sleep study. The first and currently most widely used is Type I - the comprehensive in-laboratory polysomnography, Type II - unattended comprehensive polysomnography, Type III - limited channel Pms, and Type IV monitors. But, before I start describing these methods, I have to get on my soapbox and loudly proclaim:

MEN FROM THE AGE OF FORTY AND UP AND WOMEN FROM THE AGE OF FIFTY AND UP SHOULD HAVE A SLEEP STUDY DONE ONCE EVERY FIVE YEARS.

If I could, I would shout this from the rooftops. We all have to suffer through physicals every two years after a certain age and we must endure the dreaded colonoscopy at the age of fifty, so why is it so difficult to add this one test to the list? I know what you are thinking. "How much is it going to cost me?" Or how about this thought. "I don't feel comfortable sleeping in a strange bed." Well, remember this, you could end up in a strange bed in your local hospital for much longer than one night because you never took the time to have a simple overnight sleep study.

Most insurance companies cover the cost of having either an in-lab study or the portable home sleep study. The outcome of either of the diagnostic studies will determine what mode of treatment, if any, will be followed. Which type of sleep study you are made to take is again, decided by the type of insurance that you carry and is normally of your own choosing. BUT...

If you don't enjoy being kicked out of your bedroom because you are keeping your spouse up all night or hate being made fun of by your cohorts because your snoring could wake the dead. Then decide to finally book yourself for a sleep study. If you are going into an actual lab, your appointment may be booked a few weeks out. Hopefully, you will have received the necessary paperwork beforehand. If so, then please take the time to fill it out. Normally, this should include a sleep diary. This is sent to you so the doctors have an idea of what you sleep is like in the comfort of your own home. The sleep that you get in the lab is either going to be better or worse than what you get at home, simply because, for some, it is a completely different environment and hence, uncomfortable. For others, the break from the nightly routine can be enervating, allowing them to sleep better than normal. How you react to the situation, will determine how well you sleep.

If you are having a Type I or *Comprehensive in-lab sleep study*, you will be brought to a room that will resemble a hotel room, with some labs having more lavish rooms and other labs having more basic designs. Once you settle in, you will be asked to change. A sleep technologist will come in. ask you some questions and shortly thereafter start setting you up for the study. You will be set up with wires that will similar to the image below.

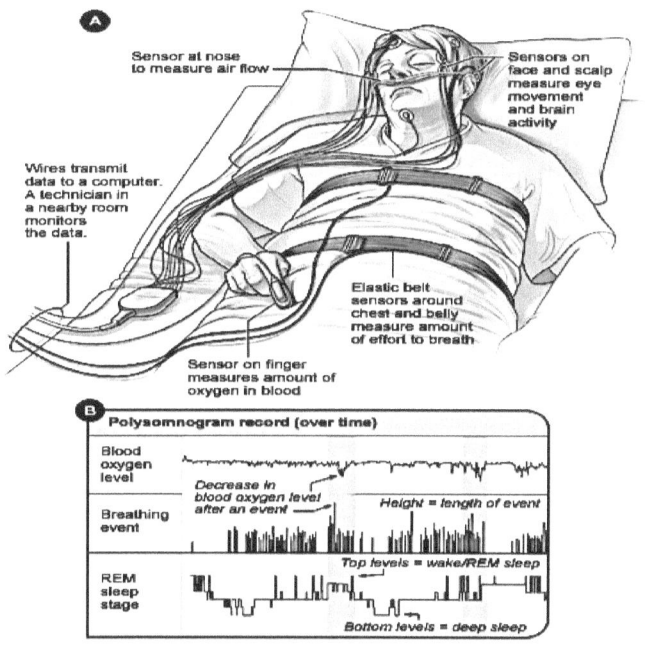

www.nih.gov

You will have wires on your head, near your eyes to help identify REM sleep, chin, neck for snoring, and legs. You will also be fitted with two belts, one around the waist and one around the chest. Last, you will have two sensors placed in front of and partly in the nose. These sensors will record the flow of air or the absence of airflow in and out of the body. These two sensors, along with the belts, are some of the most vital when diagnosing sleep apnea. The other one is the pulse/oximeter. This one records the levels of oxygen in the blood and your heart rate. I once had a patient scream out loud then burst into a giggle fit when she looked in the mirror. The cell phone comes in handy to snap a picture of yourself to show to friends and relatives. Oh yes, that happens often...

All of these wires will be connected to a box that is then connected to a cable in the wall, which, in turn, is connected to the computer that records the information. The setup normally takes approximately forty minutes. Once the setup is complete you can then read or watch television till the study starts. Lights out ranges from 10:00 to 11:00 pm. Will you feel like a puppet with all the wires attached? You very well may. Just remember, it's only for one night...at worse two nights, though not consecutively.

If you have to get up to use the bathroom, you will either call the tech or sit up on the bed and the tech will come in to disconnect you. This takes about 1 minute, since the only things that have to be disconnected are head box where all the wires are attached, the finger probe, and sometimes the cannula that looks like an oxygen tube. Once these things are disconnected, you can go merrily on your way. When you are done the tech will connect you again and you can go back to sleep. If nothing happens during the night or if you have a small number of events where you have difficulty breathing, the tech will let you sleep uninterrupted and wake you up in the morning. If it shows that you are having a significant number of events, the tech will start you on CPAP approximately two hours into the study. This is possibly the biggest advantage to the Type I monitoring; the ability to be placed on CPAP the same night. Unfortunately, this added benefit only aids those with moderate to severe sleep apnea. For those who are less severe, a second study will be needed.

CONTINUOUS POSITIVE AIRWAY PRESSURE (CPAP) is really a technical way of stating that air is being forced down your throat. Actually, it is not just air but pressurized air. Imagine sticking your head out of a moving vehicle with your mouth open; or better yet, standing in front of a fan with a funnel that covers its width and wrapping your mouth around the spout. That is CPAP. Obviously, the level of air pressure from a moving vehicle or coming from the spout is significantly stronger that what you get from CPAP. Furthermore, you are only going to get enough pressure to constantly hold your airway open while you are sleeping. CPAP is not meant to replace your own breathing. It just allows you to breathe well all night long.

If you are placed on CPAP, don't fret. Many times the brain reacts negatively to the pressurized air that the body is getting. Many times, people feel the need to breathe faster, probably to compensate for the increased pressure of the air. That will only cause possible hyperventilating. That, in turn, will cause undue stress and anxiety and the patient normally will pull the mask off the face.

Just imagine how you feel when you walk out of your house on a blustery day. Initially, it is hard to breathe but we don't go running back in the house. Instead, our brains unconsciously regulate our breathing so we can breathe in that environment. That is what you consciously have to do with CPAP. If you have difficulty exhaling against the air then take deep breaths in and exhale forcefully against the pressure. I call them *yoga breaths*. They are calming breaths. This type of deep breathing allows the brain to adapt to the pressure fairly quickly. Do this several times until your brain realizes it can breathe. Soon, you will notice that you won't be struggling that much with the flow of air. Once this happens, relax your breathing. You should be fine after that. Get comfortable and try to fall asleep again. Before you know it, the study will be over.

One small comment about the masks...there are four types... a whole face mask, full face masks, nasal masks and nasal pillows. All that will be explained in the following chapters but remember one very important thing, if you are using a nasal mask or nasal pillows, KEEP YOUR MOUTH CLOSED ALL THE TIME. If you don't do this and you open your mouth, the air will go in your nose and right out your mouth. Air, like water, will take the path of least resistance. It is easier for the air to leave a big opening like the mouth than enter a small opening like your windpipe. So keep the mouth shut. If you insist on trying it just keep in mind that you may feel like you are suffocating. Close your mouth and that sensation will go away. If you decide to try a full face mask instead, you will get the air you need no matter how you breathe.

Depending on the lab, wake up time is normally between 5:00 to 6:30 in the morning. In most labs, showers are provided though I have found that most patients prefer to go home. Please understand that if you are still feeling sleepy, report that to the tech. Coffee may be provided so that you can feel more alert on the drive home. The night tech cannot comment on the study so please do not ask. Many techs I have worked with over the years do inform their patients about the possibility of a return visit. I personally feel that it allows the patient time to acclimate to the idea of using a CPAP. Unfortunately, many patients are not made aware of their sleep apnea until they get the call to schedule the second overnight study. I personally think that it just makes an uncomfortable situation more stressful. So, my suggestion to you is to ask the tech if you may have to come back again. Hopefully you will get a yes or a no, but be happy with the maybe.

The second data collection method, Type II, is called an *unattended Comprehensive portable*. This device must have a minimum of seven channels, meaning that it must record a minimum of seven different areas. They normally are brainwaves (EEG..at least one channel), chin, snore, leads near the eyes to help identify REM, a belt for respiratory effort , heart rate (ECG), a sensor in front of the nose to record airflow and the pulse ox to record the oxygen levels. A sleep technologist or respiratory therapist normally goes to the house and sets the patient up with the system. The tech then leaves and the patient goes to sleep. In the morning a tech goes to the house to pick up the equipment. The patient is given a phone number that can be answered by the on call tech if any issues arise during the night. The accuracy of this type of study is equal to that of an in-lab study as long as the equipment functions properly during the night.

The Type III or a *limited channel Pms,* is the most common unattended home sleep test (HST) because it is significantly less complicated and comparably as accurate as an in lab study. The monitor must have a minimum of four channels.   A daytime appointment in the lab will be set up so the patient can meet with a technologist or respiratory therapist who will explain the steps to follow to do the study at home or it will be sent to the house with an explanatory DVD.   It normally consists of the two belts around the waist and the chest, a snore sensor that attached to the neck with tape, the two sensors that go in front of the nose and finally the pulse oximeter that goes on one finger. No EEG channels are used because this type of study is used mainly to record how well the patient breathes at night. In short, it records respiratory effort.

Once the patient understands the instructions, the portable monitor, along with all the monitoring sensors, will be placed in a case that will be given to the patient, or the patient will set himself or herself up at home. Once placed on the body, all the wires are connected to a monitor that is normally placed in a halter around the chest or waist. At times, the monitor may be laid at the top of the bed away from the body. It will run for one night. The patient will then take it off and return it to the lab the following day or ship it off in the mail. Most labs try to send results to the referring doctor within two weeks. If you do not hear from the doctor or the lab, please call either to get an update.

There are also less sophisticated monitoring devices available on the market called Type IV devices. They must have a minimum of 3 channels. This type of device normally records heart rate and oxygen through the pulse oximeter, a belt to record breathing effort and the cannula that sits in front of the nose to record airflow. These devices are normally worn on the wrist and monitor movement throughout the night. The accuracy is questionable, but it normally used to determine if the patient might have sleep apnea. It is not meant to diagnose the disease...only to give a preliminary assessment. This tool helps the doctor to determine what other steps should be taken to treat the patient.

CHAPTER FOUR

Do CPAP and growing old mix?

"Do not regret growing older.

It is a privilege denied to many."

Author Unknown

A while back, I was invited to give a talk about CPAP and its effect on the geriatric population. It was a disaster. It was supposed to be a show and tell presentation that turned out to be a lot more telling and not enough showing. There was another presenter who talked about inhalers and using them with the elderly. Watching her demonstrate the obstacles the elderly faced when trying to administer a dose of medication, I realized what I had done wrong. Because of that unfortunate circumstance, I was able to clearly define in my mind the hurdles my elderly patients faced when using a CPAP. Even though I worked with the elderly constantly, my response to their needs was almost automated. I was not consciously aware of the difficulties the elderly could encounter with the mask and the machine.

Several factors have to be considered when we deal with the elderly. Mobility and manual dexterity are the most important. In order to put on a mask a person has to have the ability and the strength to place a mask up and over the head. They must have the ability to rotate the arm up and behind the head in order to place the headgear on properly. Elderly patients who suffer from arthritis or rheumatism may have difficulty putting on a mask. If they are able to do so, strength is required to clip the straps in the front of the mask along with fine hand movements to maneuver the clips and adjust the Velcro straps...especially if the mask has to fit tightly to avoid leaking during the night. If a doctor requests CPAP for an elderly patient, that patient cannot suffer from any physical impairments of the upper body or a caregiver must be on hand nightly to assist the patient.

Dementia is another factor that must be taken into consideration. It is difficult enough to deal with any patient who suffers from memory loss, but adding CPAP may not be the next step. Even if an elderly patient is diagnosed with sleep apnea, it is no guarantee that CPAP will be the right choice for the patient. Again, the caregiver is ultimately the one who will determine if and when the patient will be using CPAP. If the patient wakes up disoriented and frightened because there is a strange devise attached to their face, will the caregiver have the time and patience to calm the patient down and reapply the CPAP? If this becomes a nightly ordeal, the benefit to the patient must be weighed against the psychological and physical cost placed on the caregiver and on the patient especially if this scenario is repeated more than once per night.

I have encountered many elderly patients brought in by their well-intentioned children to be screened for sleep apnea. The children talk about witnessed accounts of their parents gasping for air or breathing irregularly. Their parents normally sit quietly beside their children listening and nodding. I then ask the parents if they want to use the CPAP. Once they understand what it is and how it works, I have many respond negatively. Age becomes a factor. "I am too old for this." is a common response. I have sat in a room watching the children fret because they are worried about their parents, but many times they don't understand the time involved in getting their parent comfortable with the machine.

We all realize that learning becomes more difficult as we age. The baby boomer generation watches in amazement as their children text message with speed and accuracy. I see it with my own children. I text and it takes me a few minutes to type out a short paragraph. My sons' and daughter's response is back within moments. I am flustered by their speed and as much as I try to match them, it is useless. So imagine our parents, many who grew up when the Model T was still in production at the beginning of the industrial revolution. Try to have them text message and they will most probably walk away. As a sleep tech, I have to repeat instructions several times to many of my patients most who are from my generation or younger because they find it confusing to use a CPAP...so understand that it becomes exponentially more confusing for the elderly.

I can't help but think of my parents. My mother was diagnosed with sleep apnea several years ago. She was five feet tall and she weighed 114 lbs. when she was diagnosed. They prescribed the CPAP for her. She tried it one or two days and gave up. She placed it in her closet and after a couple of weeks, returned the unit to the company that had initially sent it to her. Afterwards, she called me and told me about her decision and I could do or say nothing that would sway her to try it again.

I look at my mother and I see a petite, beautiful, elegant, and refined woman who looks decades younger than her age and has more energy and determination than many people decades younger than her, myself included. I also consider her to be one of the most intelligent women I have ever known. Raised in Spain, she came to the United States as an adult and taught herself how to speak, read, and write English without ever attending a formal class. Her English comprehension was tested once and her command of the English language was equivalent to that of a college graduate. Yet this brilliant woman, when presented with a CPAP machine stated that it was too complicated for her. My mother's imagination has no boundaries, but computers, cell phones and any type of technology leaves her baffled. She understands that it is a necessary evil; and she realizes the interconnectivity between humanity and technology. It is just not something for her. Rest assured, she is not the only one of her generation to feel that way.

That said, there are plenty of elderly people who want to regain the vim and vigor they feel they have lost. I have had patients complain that it frustrates them that they can't seem to stay awake. For those patients, no matter what age, CPAP may be the answer. Yet I have to reiterate, some form of aid may be needed whether it be a spouse, child or professional caregiver, just to assure a proper fit. But, if all the pieces of the puzzle can fall into place; then, where there is a will, there will always be a way.

Most of the geriatric population will need a full face mask. As we age, our bodies lose the ability to regenerate as effectively as when we were younger. Our muscles become more lax, and when we fall asleep, our jaws drop open. A full face mask compensates for this by covering the both the nose and mouth. The pressurized air is delivered and the patient can breathe normally while sleeping. If the thought of a full face mask is too overwhelming, then a nasal mask with a chin strap may work. Please keep in mind it is not a jaw strap. The main function of the strap is to purse the lips together so that it is more difficult for the lips to part and allow air to escape when the patient is asleep. It is not meant to lock the upper and lower jaws together.

It is also important to note that a mask has several parts. The DME (durable medical equipment) company representative may instruct an elderly patient on disassembling and reassembling a mask for cleaning. This does not necessarily mean that the patient will fully comprehend the instructions or remember them in their entirety.

Debbie, who works as a DME rep, told me how she often encounters elderly patients who take apart the masks to clean them only to find themselves unable to put them back together. She continued by telling me how she went to an elderly patient's home because she was complaining that even though she used the machine nightly, she was still sleepy. When she asked to see the mask she realized that the patient had taken out the insert and was using the mask without it nightly because she could not put it back together. The CPAP wasn't doing anything because there was a gaping space where the insert was supposed to be; therefore, the air was just blowing in her face. This particular example reminded me how stoic the elderly are, in general. Remember that they lived through the Second World War as children or young adults. They were privy to food rationing, and when they were adults, they were subjected to the constant fear of nuclear annihilation during the Cold War. These global events changed the mindset of a generation. They are accustomed to suffering, dealing with restrictions and look upon CPAP as another circumstance that has to be endured. This poor woman told Debbie that using the CPAP was painful. She understood that her doctor wanted her to use it and she obliged even though without a cushion, the pain was severe. When Debbie met with the woman, she was confronted with a lady that had developed blisters where the hard plastic of the mask was pressing on her face. She was taught how to put the mask back together after washing and she was monitored to make sure that she had learned the technique correctly. Rest assured that this example is not the exception, but most probably the rule.

Between children, doctors, friends and relatives, the elderly are faced with an avalanche of good intentioned people all concerned with their health. It is important to remember to listen to the patient to see what they want before forcing something on them that they alone may not be able to handle.

CHAPTER FIVE

The parts of the CPAP machine

"Up your nose with a rubber hose!!"

From sitcom "Welcome back Kotter"

Once you have been diagnosed with sleep apnea, the fun begins. You will be set up with a Home care or DME (durable medical equipment) company. Who you end up with is dependent on your insurance. Many of these companies will send out a respiratory therapist to set you up with your CPAP. Others will send the machine in the mail with an enclosed DVD that will walk you through the setup. You will also receive a new mask like the one used during the sleep study, and a hose. Once everything is set up, the responsibility for maintenance, cleaning, and the replacement of worn parts shifts from the DME to you, the patient. I say this because for years, I have seen patients come into our lab complaining of resurgence of their sleepiness when all that was wrong was that the mask had worn out, or the filter was plugged or the hose was ripped, to name a few problems. THINGS WEAR OUT AND GET DIRTY. This happens with everything, so why would it not happen to everything related to your CPAP? Let's start with the parts of the CPAP and what should be done to maintain them.

The CPAP machine. The only thing you have to remember about the machine is to change the filter every three months if you have no pets and about every month if you live with pets. Regardless of any animals that share your home, it is a good idea to check the filter monthly. There may be something in your house that causes the filter to get dirty more quickly.... just change it. Use common sense. Don't wait till it is so dirty that no air is flowing through the machine or the motor fails because it is overworking trying to give you the pressure you need. Some of the filters are reusable. They look like small sponges and they can be washed with soap and water. Other filters are disposable. For example, the filters that are used on many Resmed CPAP's are disposable. They are white and yellow or white and blue. If you have a rep that tells you to flick the dust off and reuse the filter, don't do it. Let's weigh the options. Breathing in clean filtered air or using a clogged filter and possibly exposing yourself to negative health consequences because you may breathe in small particles into your lungs while on CPAP. The cost of the filter is negligible, so please call your DME representative and ask for the filters. There are many different types of machines on the market, but remember that your DME company has all of your information on file. They will know what machine you are using and they will send out the corresponding filters.

One other tidbit of information...**never, ever carry your CPAP with the water chamber filled with water**. I actually had a patient come in with his CPAP, water and all. Needless to say, the machine stopped working because the water entered the machine and ruined the motor. I called up the corresponding CPAP manufacturer and they told me that they would probably replace the machine for the patient. But, please don't count on it. Just take out the water, or better yet, don't carry the water chamber with you. It could save you future headaches and prevent disasters from happening.

The water for the water chamber.   I have come to realize that all the therapists or techs that set up patients with CPAP invariably tell the patients who they must use distilled water when using the humidifier.   NOT TRUE...Please feel free to go on the website of your CPAP manufacturer.   You will notice that when it comes to water, distilled water is recommended, but rest assured, you can use any water available to you including tap water. Though I would steer away from pond or river water.   I don't think anyone would try it, but I have witnessed stranger things than that in this business, so I decided to mention it.

The primary reason that everyone seems to be on the distilled water bandwagon is fear of damaging the water chamber. So they steer everyone away from using tap water. How that can happen is beyond me to figure out. Short of stomping on the vessel, I feel fairly confident that it is indestructible. Many patients have actually told me that they have lugged bottles of distilled water on their trips to assure themselves that they can use their humidifiers at night while away from home.   It is admirable that they do that, but it is totally unnecessary.

The major concern seems to be the accumulation of mineral deposits or unpleasant odors from well water or tap water. If that seems to be a concern, here are some solutions. For those nasty mineral deposits, just soak the water chamber in white vinegar and it should dissolve the deposits in about an hour. (The proportions of white vinegar to water are 3 to 1 or one third is vinegar and two thirds is water.)   As far as smells are concerned, chlorine, which is added to municipal or city water, will dissipate very quickly if you just fill a jug with water and let it sit for a short period of time before putting it in your water chamber. The chlorine molecule is very volatile when exposed to air so it will leave the water if you give the container a couple of shakes before using your humidifier. Other people use bottled water. Just remember that the Environmental Protection Agency (EPA) governs city water; if you have access to it. Bottled water is considered a "food", therefore, it is governed by the Food and Drug Administration (FDA). The EPA has much stricter guidelines for water treatment than the FDA. Moreover, the EPA requires that city residents be provided with a detailed list stating the origin of the water and what, if any contaminants are in the water. The FDA has no such requirements.

Bottled water also costs more, and causes more waste in landfills because of the plastic bottles that are used to deliver the water. So, yes, I would like you to be greener when using CPAP. I remember drinking water from the water fountain when I was growing up till it became an "uncool" thing to do. None of us suffered any side effects because we drank water in that manner and probably, even today, the water would still quench our thirst just as effectively. But, if the idea of using bottled water is more appealing, please invest in a filter for your sink. You will get better results and the same bottled water feel without all the extra plastic and expense. All details pertaining to the differences between tap and bottled water can be found at the website

Allaboutwater.org.

It is definitely eye opening and a must read. Well then, now that I have touted the benefits of using tap water, some of you may say...but my water stinks! The only time that I personally remember water having a pungent odor was when I lived in Florida. When those sprinklers were running I could smell the "lovely" odor of rotten eggs for miles. The compound known as hydrogen sulfide was the culprit that produced that odiferous aroma. It is a product of decaying organic matter in the ground. This odor also permeated the house my son and his housemates rented when he was living off campus while going to college in Connecticut. When he and his friends first moved into the house they were assailed with the strong odor when they ran the water. They mentioned it to their landlord and he calmly stated that he had lived there for years and as long as the water was used daily, the odor would eventually go away.   That is exactly what happened.   But if you are constantly fighting this battle, then use distilled or bottled water. If the sulfur smell comes from the hot water, have your hot water heater checked.

One thing that I do want to clarify is this; **the vapor that you are breathing in while on CPAP is actually distilled water.** For those of you who don't remember your Chemistry, distilled water is made from the steam collected from boiling water. So except for issues with odors, it really doesn't matter where the water comes from. The steam (water vapor) is all that is going into those precious lungs. So, in short, keep the chamber clean. If all else fails, just call your home care company and have them send you a new one. Most of the water chambers are covered by insurance so there should be no out of pocket expense or at the most, a very minimal one.

The humidifier. That is the part of the CPAP that regulates the amount of water vapor you will breathe in during the night. If you have a heated humidifier you will have a knob of some sort with numbers or roman numerals at each notch. This knob is normally on the top of the CPAP above the place where you insert your container. The level of evaporation is regulated by this knob. This increases or decreases the heating plate at the base of the water chamber. The higher the number the more humidity is produced.

YOU CAN NEVER GET TOO MUCH HUMIDITY. You want to wake up and feel like you do in the daytime. You do not want to wake up with your tongue stuck to the roof of your mouth and you do not want to have to wake up at night to get a drink of water. If this is happening, then something is wrong. Increase your humidity level to see if that fixes the problem.

<u>LISTEN TO YOUR BODY</u>. It will tell you what it needs. It will tell you when it is getting too much by rejecting the excess humidity being provided by the water chamber. This will manifest itself through excess water in the mask or a pool of water in your mouth when you wake up. You will probably have to remove your mask to shake out the water. At times, the excess water travels down the hose. I actually had a young man who came into the lab for a CPAP titration. I started the study with heated humidification. I entered a couple of hours later because the patient was complaining of getting too much moisture. When I went to check his mask I noticed that the air pressure had decreased. I took the mask and the hose off to remove the excess water. When I went to the sink to shake the hose, I was surprised by a large quantity of water that poured out. Once I dried off everything, I placed the mask back on the patient and immediately lowered the heat level to "0" but I still left water in the chamber. He was now getting what is known as passover humidity. It is very similar to the residual moisture you feel when standing near a lake or the ocean. A current of air that flows over the water produces it. It picks up some moisture simply because as the air is flowing it is in contact with the water. It is not a lot of moisture, but for some, it is sufficient as was exemplified by this patient. He woke up feeling fine the following morning. So, if this happens to you, don't be afraid to lower the heat level.

A gurgling sound in your hose could also be caused by something known as rainout. This is caused when the air surrounding the hose is colder than the air inside the hose. It is more commonly known as condensation. To prevent the condensation, buy a CPAP hose sock. They can readily be found on the internet at a very reasonable cost. Better yet, buy a scrap of material (I recommend fleece or something similar) and sew it to form a tube. Add elastic at either end to keep it on the hose and you will have made your own sock for your hose. It's a lot cheaper and you can choose the material that suits your fancy. Many of my patients get around that by just keeping the hose under the covers. This works if you don't tend to move around too much in bed. If you change positions often, opt for the sock.

For people who are well hydrated, the level of humidity will probably be low. If, on the other hand, you are taking water pills, or any medication that can cause excessive dry mouth, the level of humidity from the humidifier will be more. This level will also change with the seasons. In northern climates this is especially true. In the summer, because of the increased humidity in the air, you could probably get away with a low heat setting or have the setting at zero. Some patients never use the humidifier. Remember that the body is highly adaptable. So, if you have gotten used to using the CPAP without the humidifier, then you will probably not want to ever incorporate it. That is fine. If, on the other hand you are new to CPAP, you will normally be supplied with an integrated humidifier. This will give you the option to try using your CPAP in a variety of ways.

Normally, I suggest that patients try the humidifier from the onset. The lungs are warm and moist. So, does it not sound logical to give the body what it is accustomed to getting? The noses that sit in the middle of our faces are not there for decorative reasons; nor are they there to give us our distinctive personalities. So when starting on CPAP it could be reasonably assumed that we should get warmed and moistened air from our CPAPs. It actually helps the body adjust to using a CPAP more quickly if the humidity is used; but ultimately, the decision to use the humidifier rests in your hands. If you do decide to use the humidifier, remember one thing...

PLAY WITH THE HUMIDITY LEVEL ON YOUR MACHINE. Adjust the settings as the seasons change depending on how you feel and notice if there is any change in mouth dryness or if you are ever placed on a different drug than any you have previously taken. If you do this, you will eventually learn what works for you and your sleep will be better at night. Go up or down one level and judge the outcome the following morning. Within a few days you should be able to reach your optimal level.

CHAPTER SIX

So what is the best mask for me?

*We will take our masks off that we use at night to live our
lives with purpose throughout the day*

Modified from a quote from Kimberly Cohe

I mentioned earlier that there are four types of masks
on the market. The whole face mask, full face masks, nasal
masks and nasal pillows. I will start from the smallest and
progress to the largest. But before we start I have to go
back to the issue of the air pressure. If you have been privy
to an infant's reaction to gusty winds when the child is
taken outside you will appreciate and understand what
your brain is doing to you. For those of you who have
never seen this I will elaborate. The nervous system of an
infant is obviously new. It has to learn from every
experience it encounters. So, when the brain is presented
with that gust of wind it has never before encountered, the
child becomes startled. That is a reaction to the shock of
the new experience, but we as parents, aunts, uncles, etc.
do not grab that infant and run back inside; we instead,
stay and go about our business, possibly cooing at the
baby or chuckling at the startled reaction simply because
most anything an infant does is generally cute.

That reaction is generated by the autonomic nervous
system. It regulates all visceral functions (ie., digestion,
heart rate, salivation, etc.) within the body including
breathing. When you put on a CPAP mask for the first

49

time, the autonomic nervous system may react in the same way as that of the infant's. I recommend doing what I call YOGA BREATHS. No matter what mask you have on, take deep breaths in and out slowly. If you are using nasal pillows or nasal masks, this breathing must only be done in and out through the nose. If you have the full face or whole face mask, it doesn't matter how you breathe as long as you continue to breathe in this manner till your autonomic nervous system realizes that it can breathe normally against the pressurized air. Once you start feeling comfortable with the air, relax your breathing. Your goal is not to hyperventilate, but to breathe. You may have to repeat this technique over the course of several evenings as you start using your CPAP until your body becomes accustomed to the airflow. Once this happens you will have become desensitized to the force of the air. At that point, the Yoga Breaths will be unnecessary.

Nasal Pillows

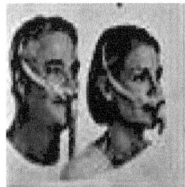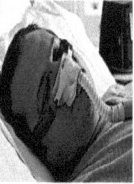

Nasal pillows are the least intrusive masks available. A nasal pillow mask fits just under the nose and seals up the nares or nostrils completely, thus allowing the air to travel from the machine directly into the throat. Patients who read or watch television in bed normally use this type of mask. It is also the most attractive of the masks available on the market. It also seems to work best with patients who are on lower pressures. It has been my mainstay for people who suffer from claustrophobia. Because the mask sits below a person's line of vision, it normally does not trigger a panic attack when the patient has it on. Over time, a person becomes desensitized to using the mask. It is at this point that other masks can be tried if the nasal pillows are too uncomfortable, although I tend to think that it is one of the most popular types of masks on the market. The pillows, or the part that sits in the nostrils, comes in different sizes; extra small, small, medium and large. These sizes fit approximately 90% to 95% of the population. Unfortunately at present, there are no larger sizes to fit larger noses, but don't despair...I am sure that it won't take long for that minor issue to be resolved.

Some of my patients have complained that they seem to get too much air when they are using the nasal pillows. Most of them state that they have difficulty breathing out against the air. This sensation is due to the fact that the air travels up the CPAP hose and directly into the nasal passages. I compare the sensation to standing in a wind tunnel with the air blowing straight at you or better yet, having two jet engines blowing air up your nose. Some people develop sores or scabs inside the nose from the pressure. This could be due to a lack of humidity or that the nose is pressure sensitive. It seems that the force of the airflow can, at times, irritate the nasal tissue. Many times this issue can be resolved by increasing the humidity levels (temperature) or by using a nasal moisturizing gel. There are several on the market but to make sure that you are getting the best one, please ask a pharmacist to recommend a brand that is water soluble. Please, **never, ever** use Vaseline or Vicks in your nose when using your CPAP. It is true that they help to lubricate the nasal passageways; but they are petroleum (oil) based products.

Our bodies consist of about 75% water and as is common knowledge that oil and water don't mix. The air pressure of the machine will force the petroleum particles deep into the lungs where they will get trapped and may never get out. Why open yourself up to a possible infection. Enough said…

Nasal Masks

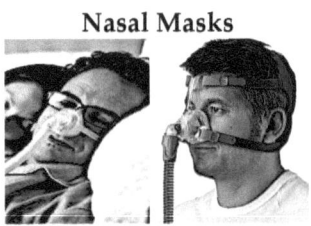

The next type of mask on the market is the nasal mask. It covers the entire nose. It is shaped in the form of a triangle with a head strap that wraps around your forehead and another one that runs around the head and under the earlobes. Some of the masks have a gel or cushion insert and others are made solely from double-layered silicone. They work very well with the vast majority of patients and for most no problems arise. Many people prefer this type of mask to the nasal pillows because the way the air is delivered is not as direct. It travels up the hose, hits the face and bounces back into the mask forming a zone of air turbulence. The body can then draw the air from this with each breath. Even though the difference between the delivery of the air through the nasal masks is minutely slower than that of the nasal pillows, the brain can tell the difference. The air through the nasal masks seems to be more tolerable for many CP AP users, because it doesn't feel as forced. Just remember, that the body adapts to all sorts of conditions. Just give yourself time and you will be able to adjust to any circumstance. In all the years of working with patients using CPAP, I only came across one patient who could not tolerate the air. This surprised him because he stated that he wore a gas mask at work almost every day. The difference was that the mask he used obviously only supplied him with filtered air, not pressurized filtered air. I honestly do not think that he was ever able to overcome his feeling of panic when the air was turned on. This again exemplifies how different every individual can be and how differently everybody can react to using CPAP. But please don't fret; in all probability, you will be able to adapt to CPAP with no major issues.

Full Face Masks

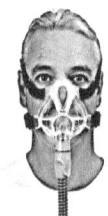 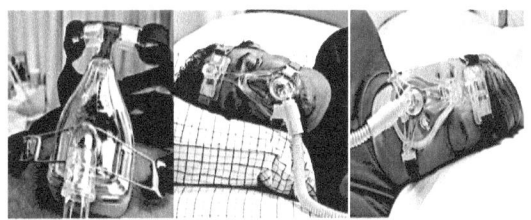

A full face masks covers the nose and the mouth. It looks like a large triangular mask with the same type of headgear as the nasal masks and fitting around the head in the same manner. These masks are used under several circumstances, the most common being a patient who is a mouth breather. Many times patients have come into my lab stating that they sleep with their mouth open. This doesn't necessarily mean that they are mouth breathers. If there are no chronic sinus issues, or constant problems with nasal allergies or even having a deviated septum, I tend to try a nasal mask first. Since the surface area is smaller, the seal tends to be better. If I have a patient who suffers from the aforementioned maladies, I will fit the patient with a full face mask. This allows the wearer to breathe through the nose or the mouth. If you opt to use the full face mask, humidification will probably play an important part in improving the length of time you are on CPAP during the night because the saliva in your mouth will do nothing to help you avoid feeling parched like the Sahara. Saliva plays an important role in digesting our food. It is chock full of enzymes that start breaking down food particles before they proceed to the stomach. Saliva is not meant to warm and moisten the air that you breathe in. Our noses were designed for that singular purpose, as previously stated in an earlier chapter.

Our noses have turbinates that are covered with small hairs or cilia. These cilia are, in turn, covered in mucus that helps add moisture to the air we inhale as well as acting like a filter and trapping any unsavory particles that try to invade our bodies. Between the two, the air is surrounded, cleaned and prepared for the lungs. When using a CPAP with a full face mask, the hepa filter at the back of the machine and the humidifier in the front preform the same function. Full face masks also come with gel or foam inserts or they can be clear. They have knobs that turn to adjust the angle of the mask on the face or hinges that perform the same function. Both of these are located parallel to the bridge of the nose.

The Whole Face Mask seals the face within the mask. The interface runs along the surface of the bone starting from the forehead down the sides near the hairline to the jaw and forward to the chin. This is another mask that seems to work well with people who suffer from claustrophobia. It works because once the mask is on the face it is visually unobtrusive and looking through the mask is analogous to looking through a window. To clarify, yes, the eyes are inside the mask. Most of my patients, who use this mask, state that their eyes do not dry out with the air.

Total Face Masks

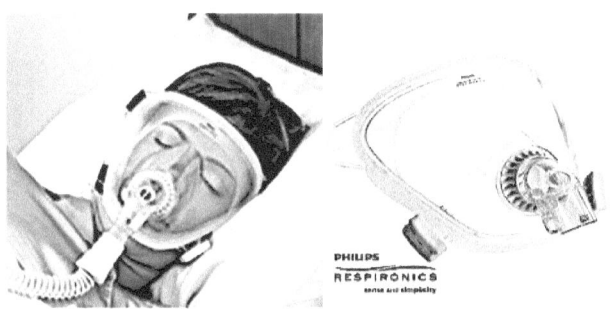

Respironics Fit Life Whole Face Mask

This particular mask comes in only two sizes... small and large. The small size would probably fit children or very petite women. The large is made more for the general adult population. I have had patients compare this mask to the ones used by fighter pilots. Get ready for liftoff!!! This is another very common comment. But, if it works for you that is all that really matters. So you can fall asleep thinking that you are a fighter pilot. Maybe one day you will wake up with so much energy that you may think that it could become a reality. Stranger things have happened.

CHAPTER SEVEN

Cleaning and maintaining the equipment

What separates two people most profoundly is a different sense and degree of cleanliness

Freidrich Nietxche

I have been in the field of sleep for many years and it still amazed at how often I see patients using a CPAP that is filthy! I cannot fathom how oblivious people are to the actual function of the CPAP. My candid observation was further affirmed when I heard many of my patients referring to their machine as a "CPAK". I always wondered how that name was derived. There was a movie in 2001 called K-PAX with Kevin Spacey about an alien being who came to earth. Could that be the origin? Using a CPAP could seem scifi-ish to some; so much so that quite a few of my patients refused to use it. Or maybe it was similar to singing the lyrics to our favorite songs. I remember injecting similar sounding words to many songs I sang as I enjoyed the music simply because I didn't understand what was being sung. That didn't deter me. I wanted to sing and I would do that no matter how odd it sounded. Sometimes, I was actually disappointed when I finally did find out the actual lyrics simply because I liked my version better. Maybe this innocent oblivion has been carried over to the machine. It could also be the reason that many ignored the necessity of maintaining their equipment.

So let me go back to the basics. A CPAP is a machine that is forcing air down the throat so a person with sleep apnea can breathe. It is pushing the forced air or Air Pressure continuously, hence:

Continuous Positive Air Pressure

If the machine is not cleaned properly, along with that air, dust, pollen and even mold can be carried into the machine through the motor and eventually maybe even into the lung.

We have all seen pictures of dust mites and all the other creepy crawlies that share our living space. They are ugly little things and the thought that I have to share my life with many of them gives me the willies. Conversely, I personally think that eating dirt when you are a child is a good thing. It helps build our immune system (not that I ever fed dirt to my children; but I am sure that they sampled that and many other weird things when they were growing up). Does this mean that I will allow my patients to go merrily along with their lives unaware of the dangers that they may be facing? I most certainly will not. I reiterate, we are talking about forced air when we are talking about CPAP. Besides damaging the motor, forcing anything down into the lungs is equivalent to playing Russian roulette with your health. I would never put anyone in a wind tunnel filled with dust bunnies, ask them to open their mouths and turn on the turbines. That would be insane! So please tell me, what is the difference when a CPAP is turned when no filters are in place or the filters on the machine are dirty?

I recall a patient who came into the lab complaining that the CPAP had lost pressure. He was feeling sleepy again and he wondered if his machine was malfunctioning. The tech looked at the machine and turned it on. Sure enough, very little air was coming out, yet the motor sounded as if it was straining. He turned the machine around to look at the filter. It was in place but it was almost black it was so dirty. So the tech proceeded to take out the filter. He turned the CPAP on again and a puff of dust blew out of the machine, which surprised the tech and the patient. The motor was then able to work properly which allowed the air to flow through the machine unhindered. This patient had been on CPAP for years and had never replaced the filter. In defense of all of you who have done the same, I understand. It must be disconcerting to have a strange person walk nonchalantly into your home and place this odd machine on the nightstand. You stand there confused and bewildered as this person proceeds to connect all the cables, fit you with a mask and quickly explain what button to push to start up everything. Many patients who I have talked to have told me that the rep states clearly that they should not touch anything other than the on-off button because all the demons in hell will come down and bear the weight of their fury upon them, the world will end, and chaos will ensue...In other words, they know what your body needs and you should not change ANYTHING.

I am here to tell you that this is not the case. You must be proactive when it comes to your CPAP. In the same manner that you maintain a car so it will last you a while, you must care for that machine that is occupying space on your nightstand. If you treat it with kindness, it will return

59

the favor by helping you achieve a better quality of life.

First, look at the back of the machine and find the filter. Your filter will be unique to your CPAP based on the specifications of the manufacturer of your machine. Some are disposable and some are reusable. Your DME provider will be able to tell you which type fits your machine.

Types of CPAP filters

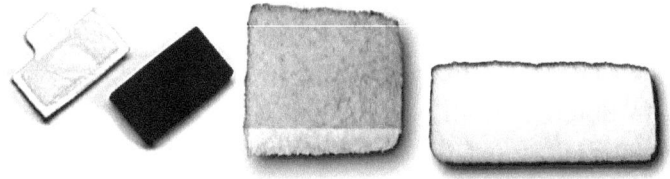

If you have pets, it is advisable that you check your filter monthly because pet dander and fur may obstruct the flow of the air. Otherwise, a filter should last about three months. Think of how the machine works. The air is being sucked into the machine in the same manner that a vacuum cleaner sucks up dirt from your floors. It's that suction that allows you to clean your house. In a vacuum cleaner the filter is at the end where the air exits the machine. In this way, the dirt is not reintroduced back into your house but stays in the receptacle. With a CPAP the inverse is true. The filter is located at the entrance of the machine so the air that you breathe is filtered and clean.

Dust the top of the CPAP every time you dust. It will help to maintain the overall appearance of the machine. I have another patient who is diligent about cleaning her CPAP. She is elderly and she frets about the possible physical damage she may suffer if her CPAP is not clean. It frightens her to think that she could expose herself to unwarranted infections due to a minor lapse in CPAP maintenance. It was this fear that prompted her to come to see me about a minor issue involving her machine. She handed the case over to me and I opened it up to reveal its contents. Her mask was protected with the original packaging because she was afraid about germs attacking her if she let it lie. She explained how diligent she was about maintaining her equipment yet when I lifted her machine from the bag I noticed it was encrusted with gunk. She clearly followed my instructions and those of the DME representative to the letter. Internally, her machine ran as smoothly as the first day she used it several years earlier. Her mask was perfect and her hose looked like new. As I looked at her machine, I begin to ponder how it had arrived at this state. Did she eat near it? Was her house clean? Did her grandchildren run cookie filled hands over the top trying to unravel the mystery of her CPAP? My curiosity nibbled at my mind as I helped her with minor issues. She told me that she loved it and she used it nightly. Her children told me she was a new woman. So if she loved it so much, why not wipe the top to keep it clean. I later found out that she didn't do it because she was never instructed to do so. It was then that I realized that sometimes things that are self-explanatory to me my not be so for other people. The water chamber should be washed out and left open to air dry about once a week. White vinegar works wonders. It is a natural antiseptic and antibacterial when used full strength. It is also an environmentally green product. If you use well water, the vinegar will remove the mineral deposits and leave your water chamber like new. If you don't like the smell, rinse the container with some liquid dish soap diluted in water. Just make sure that you are using a product that is NOT antibacterial. Rinse out the chamber till the soap has been completely removed. Some water chambers are dishwasher safe as long as they are put on the top rack. If you are not sure, call the manufacturer or the DME provider and they will be able to tell you.

I have had patients tell me that they have followed my instructions or those of the DME provider and mold has still grown in the water chamber. This normally happens to people who go to warmer climates where the humidity levels in the air are naturally higher. Even though the manufacturers recommend not using bleach, I will still encourage you to do so. Just make sure that the correct proportions of water and bleach needed to disinfect surfaces are followed exactly as printed on the label of the bleach container. It will effectively kill the mold and bacteria and it can easily be removed by rinsing out well with water. Just make sure that the bleach does not sit in the chamber for more than 10 minutes since the corrosive nature of bleach will interact with the metal at the base of the chamber and it may begin to eat away at it. If this does happen, do not fret. Just call your DME provider and they should be able to send you a new one. They can normally be replaced every six months if necessary.

Disconnect the hose from your CPAP daily and drape it over a door. I would love it if everyone would rinse out his or her hose after it was disconnected, but I understand that we do not live in a perfect world. As long as air it permitted to run through the hose during the day, that should allow whatever residual moisture to evaporate.

Even if it does not do so, it will help to prevent bacteria and odors to build up in the hose. If possible, wash the hose often. Daily, weekly, or monthly…just do it. Your mask is another very important part of your therapy. Most masks last about six months. If you have oily skin, I recommend that you become more vigilant about maintaining your mask. The oils and salts from the skin tend to degrade the mask more quickly. Another problem with oily skin is that the oils start to build up on the surface of the mask. This, in turn, causes the surface of the mask to become slicker, which will cause the mask to slide on the skin as a person sleeps causing leaks, discomfort and at times pain. Take your mask in hand and face it towards you as if you were about to put it on. Run your finger over the surface that is normally in contact with your skin. If your finger slides easily over the surface, you have an oily buildup on the surface of the mask. This is also true for women who use lotions on their face before retiring for the night. Wash the mask with warm soapy water, preferably using a mild dish soap, till all the oils are removed.

I have encouraged many of my patients to take the mask with them into the shower, but not the headgear. Since most people take showers in the morning it, kills two birds with one stone. The mask is cleaned along with the rest of you and it eliminates an extra step as far as maintaining the mask. Once done, air dry on a counter or over a hook or door. Make sure to frequently wash the ends of the hose that connect to the mask and the CPAP machine. I have noticed that oils accumulate in these areas especially for people with oily complexions, causing the hose to slip off. It is rare, but it does occur. Vigilance is the key with successful CPAP use. Be aware of any changes and ask for help. Better to seek a solution than struggle in the darkness, literally.

CHAPTER EIGHT

Problems with CPAP

Oh that all my troubles would disappear and I could relish daily the joys of life, yet constantly I am plagued by minor issues that cloud my temperament and sour my days.

Elizabeth Lowe

Over time, I have witnessed many problems arising from using a CPAP mask. Some patients love the mask when they are placed on CPAP the first night but at home they have a hard time keeping the mask on for long periods. They fret and become anxious about using the machine to the point that they decide it is not worth the stress and they give up. The CPAP ends up in the closet stuffed away and eventually forgotten. Following is a list of the most common issues that arise while using CPAP.

Rhinitis

I remember a patient who tolerated using his CPAP after I "scared him to death" about the suffering endured by the body when good sleep is not achieved nightly. He decided to go with the nasal pillows because he didn't want to deal with a larger mask. After using the CPAP for a short time, he started to develop cold like symptoms that were more pronounced when he woke up in the morning. He would have to blow his nose several times and suffer through a stuffy nose that could last several hours. He admitted that he felt better with the CPAP but the daily nasal discomfort was becoming aggravating. Since he was a practicing attorney, it was imperative that he could present his cases in court without the aid of a box of tissues at his side. He called me in desperation and I explained that he probably was suffering from a rare side effect caused by his CPAP. The symptoms most resemble those of a cold. Runny noses and pressure behind the eyes are the most common complaint. The constant air pressure flowing up through the nasal passage may cause these cold-like symptoms. With some patients, this constant airflow can cause the nasal passageways to become irritated and thereby become inflamed. With other patients it is the coldness of the air that is the culprit. The doctor may prescribe an antihistamine or nasal decongestant along with varying the humidity levels. Most of the time, increasing the humidity helps; but for some, the increased humidity only makes things worse. Trying a larger mask can, at times, help decrease this irritation because the delivery of the air is less forceful. The air pressure is the same; it just does not feel like it is being delivered by two turbine jet engines for lack of a better analogy. With a nasal mask or a full face mask, the air is more dispersed throughout the mask allowing the body to draw the air in with each breath instead of having it forced up the nose. This occurs when the air travels up the hose, hits the face and bounces back into the back of the mask causing turbulence. The body then breathes off of this turbulent air in the mask. Though it is only a few milliseconds of difference, the brain and the nasal tissue sense the difference and may respond more favorably to the less forceful method of delivery. Nasal congestion or irritation may also be triggered by not being vigilant about changing the filter, though that seems to be the least common contributor to this condition. As this patient was very diligent about maintaining his CPAP, the above did not apply to him. He had no interest in changing to a larger mask because he felt it was more "unattractive" and since he had accepted the fact that a CPAP was going to be a part of maintaining a healthy lifestyle, he wanted to look as good as possible while using it. He came in to see one of our doctors and he was prescribed prescription nasal decongestants. The medication did improve his rhinitis significantly though not entirely. He eventually did try a nasal mask and he would alternate between the pillows and the mask. This technique helped reduce his discomfort to the point that using his CPAP became tolerable.

Those "lovely" skin abrasions

Another very common occurrence is the appearance of a sore or welt on the bridge of the nose. For those that use the nasal mask, a quick fix could be changing over to a nasal pillow interface. The pictures on page 31 show how the nasal pillows completely by-pass the affected area. This type of mask also allows the wearer to read, watch television and if the need should arise allows the patient to use the restroom without having to remove the mask.

If this type of mask is uncomfortable, (some people cannot tolerate having something in their nares) then a nasal mask is the only other alternative. I have had the misfortune of having to deal with many of my patients who suffer nightly trying to alleviate the pain that develops over the course of the evening. Many use Band-Aids, to protect the areas most affected. Others use gauze, tissues, and any other thing that they can lay their desperate hands upon to help resolve the problem. One of the products that I recommend is Dr. Scholl's Moleskin. It is normally found in your local pharmacy in the section that deals with foot products. It is made of a felt like material on one side and an adhesive on the other side. Some patients fold the adhesive portion in on itself so that all that can be seen is the moleskin. They then cut strips wide enough to cover the affected area. One strip is then placed on the bridge of the nose and the mask rests over it. The moleskin acts as a buffer between the interface or the surface of the mask and the skin on the nose. For many, this works very well.

Case in point, a very sweet patient of mine who is a great advocate of CPAP, came in to see me because she was having a minor issue with her mask. She proceeded to take out her full face mask and show it to me. Her mask was a Mirage Quattro with a clear silicone cushion. I noticed that her cushion was covered with a layer of moleskin. She stated that the moleskin had helped her eliminate the constant irritation that she struggled with on the top of her nose. She was pleased and grateful with my suggestion, but she stated that this particular mask was causing her discomfort. As I examined her mask, I looked at her ingenious application of the moleskin in wonder because using it in that particular manner had not occurred to me. I was further impressed by the fact that for her, this method actually worked. Her issue was resolved when she was fitted with a smaller mask, since the DME provider had inadvertently sent her the wrong size when they had shipped out her replacement. SIZE MATTERS!!!! Especially with your masks, so please check that the correct size is delivered to you.

Another aid on the market that helps patients who suffer from constant soreness is the Comfort Care Pad. It is a gel filled pad that rests on the bridge of the nose and under the mask providing a buffer between your skin and the silicone of the mask. It comes in two sizes and there is no adhesive on the pad because the pressure of the mask on the face is meant to keep the pad in place. I have had patients who have had great success with this and others that have not. It is something that will be based entirely on personal preference and level of comfort.

Remzzzs **(http://www.remzzzs.com)** is a company that sells CPAP liners for those suffering from CPAP woes. They have developed an all-natural product that sits on top of the silicone interface and helps to seal the mask to the face. These can be used with nasal masks or with full face. They are meant to be disposable because the liners are designed to absorb the oils and perspiration that can cause irritation during the night. If cost is a concern, the liners can be used more than once, though it is recommended that the liners be changed out nightly. The company has been around for approximately 5 years. Their dedicated website offers more detailed information with a toll free number that you can call with any questions.

So you can try them out and decide for yourself if it is something that will make CPAP more comfortable during the night. Remzzzs are also covered by most insurance plans. To find out how insurance reimbursement works, please feel free to contact the company directly or call your DME provider. They are also compatible with a varied assortment of masks manufactured by Fisher & Paykel, Respironics and ResMed.

Pad-a-Cheek (www.padacheek.com) is another company that makes CPAP mask liners. A woman diagnosed with sleep apnea, who suffered from the same nightly maladies, formed the company in 2004. The company sells a variety of fleece covers for CPAP masks and the headgear to help reduce pressure and minimize the skin irritation that many times is associated with wearing CPAP. The covers made from polyester, are offered in a variety of colors and are also machine washable.

As with anything, it all comes down to personal preference. Try all the liners out if need be, to find the one that best suits your needs. Necessity is the mother of invention and as always, new products to combat CPAP or make using the machine more comfortable, will abound.

Dryness

Nightmares of roaming the Sahara deprived of water seem to creep into the subconscious when this topic is mentioned. Yes, many of the veteran CPAP users do not feel the need for humidification when using their machine, For newbies, I have discovered that it is a useful tool to help acclimate a patient sooner to their new best friend. We are warm and moist on the inside, so it stands to reason that the air that enters the body is more readily used by the body if it is delivered in that manner. Our noses were designed over eons to filter out foreign particulates and prepare the air before it enters our lungs. CPAP, especially the older models, did not have a water chamber. For years, CPAP delivered pressurized air and nothing else. Eventually, humidifiers were incorporated, but they were cold. That actually exacerbated the nasal discomfort by making the air significantly colder. As many of you have noticed, air gets colder when it circulates or moves. Add cold water to that and patients were breathing in the equivalent of arctic air when they used their machines. Needless to say, many discarded the water chambers and even their CPAPs in disgust. With the advent of warm humidification those that strayed started to attempt using their machines again. For the majority, that was a welcome addition. Yet many users still faced obstacles that needed to be overcome. The hows of using a heated humidifier was the biggest stumbling block…such an easy premise with so many variants.

I reiterate. LISTEN TO YOUR BODY. If the body needs water, it will send the signal for you to drink. It will continue to send that signal till that need is satisfied. A funny thing about thirst is that it is often times confused with hunger. Could it be that many of those "cravings" that we have are actually our brains telling us that we need water? Amazingly, this happens to us quite often throughout the day and even at night. If the body is dehydrated, it will look for water. If a CPAP is using a low level of humidity, the brain will try to get more moisture from the machine. When it cannot, it will open the mouth in the hopes that it will be able to get that moisture from the environment. What then happens is that a huge leak forms, especially if the patient is using nasal pillows or nasal masks. The patient wakes up parched and annoyed stating that they keep on opening their mouth while on CPAP. A simple solution could just be increasing the level of humidity by turning the knob up a notch.   Then the opposite can occur where too much humidity is being delivered. To some, it may feel as if one is the unfortunate victim of self-imposed waterboarding. Though there may

be the sudden urge to pull the mask off
while fighting the increased water bubbling up your hose and run screaming into the night, fear not. Your body is just telling you that it is getting too much of a good thing. Even though our bodies are 75% water, sometimes our bodies are sufficiently hydrated that any extra water is not welcomed. Adjust the humidity level down and that should easily fix the problem. Medications, overexertion or simply not drinking enough liquids can contribute to an increased need for humidity. I can personally vouch for the fact that in many instances this simple change was the difference between a compliant patient and a patient who could not tolerate the CPAP. We do not give our bodies the credit they deserve. Our bodies try to tell us what we need and when we do not deliver, it compensates for what it is missing. Generally our bodies are very forgiving but even our bodies have their limits.

Aerophagia, or the swallowing of air.

At times this can happen with patients. It seems that the brain has difficulty adjusting to the   constant   pressure that is being delivered to the body. Many times this happens when the patient is sleeping laterally or on his/her side. The air that is used by the body to keep the airway open when sleeping on the back cannot be exhaled properly when the person is sleeping on his or her side. Since the excess air has nowhere to go, it is swallowed. This can cause bloating, belching and a general feeling of discomfort. Some of my patients have stated that it takes several hours to rid the body of this excess air.

Chipmunk cheeks!!!

These normally occur with full face masks. Most patients who use these types of masks actually are mouth breathers. Allergies, chronic sinus issues, a deviated septum, age, or a combination of these factors can be reason enough to opt for a full face mask. The inflated cheeks occur when the air from the hose enters the mouth. Our mouths are designed to receive food and liquids. They are meant to be pliable for this reason.

Children seem to have fun sticking their faces out the car window and opening their mouths to let the air that is rushing past flow in. They giggle at the sensation they get when this happens...very similar to becoming a blowfish. Once they have had enough, they stick their heads back in the car and continue on to other forms of entertainment no worse for the wear. The air from you machine is acting in the same manner as the air flowing past the car. It fills the inside of your mouth but instead of giggling, you stress because you feel as if the air has nowhere to go. This is normal. If possible, close your mouth and breathe through your nose. If you simply can't, a chinstrap may help in preventing the cheeks from puffing out. This would be worn in conjunction with the full face mask. Another way to resolve this minor discomfort is by increasing the EPR or Flex mode on your machine if your machine comes equipped with either of those functions. Most of the newer machines have this option. This would allow the air to back off more when you exhaled minimizing the secondary effects of the excess air. If all else fails, increase the humidity one more notch so that the mouth does not dry out and imagine yourself as that child again.

The blasted air itself!!!

No pun intended, but yes, the force of the air can be a big detriment to using a CPAP. I have already explained that using yoga breaths, as I call them, help to give your brain time to adjust to the flow of the air. Another very popular method is using the CFlex or EPR mode on your CPAPs. Respironics machines have the flex mode with their newer models. ResMed uses EPR (expiratory pressure relief). Both allow an ebbing and flowing of the air as you breathe. This means that you will get the full pressure that you need when you inhale the air but the pressure will back off as you exhale or breathe out your air. It is a great tool to allow the body to get comfortable with using a CPAP. Remember that you may be gung ho about using a CPAP, but your sleeping brain may be totally against it. That is why it is important to give your body time. It does seem that I am splitting you into two entities? In a sense, I am. Your sleeping brain or the autonomic nervous system, acts very differently than your conscious brain. You can rationalize and decipher the things that affect your life. You can interpret actions or circumstances that affect your life daily and act upon them with full knowledge of why you have chosen that action. Your sleeping brain never will.

Over-titration is a fairly common occurrence in some labs. Some sleep techs are overzealous when it comes to increasing pressure on a patient. If they see that the patient is having some residual waxing and waning of their breathing, they can increase the pressure to compensate instead of allowing the brain to adjust to the air pressure. Bringing up the pressure one or two centimeters of water pressure is not gravely erroneous, but if the pressure increases significantly, then problems can occur. The after effects on some patients can be interrupted sleep patterns and continued drowsiness. If, after being on CPAP for month or two, you find that it is still difficult for you to keep the mask on and you are struggling with the air pressure, over titration could be the culprit. Call your lab and ask if it is possible to have your pressure settings checked. The first thing that the lab would probably do is order a download of your usage data. The data is transferred from your machine onto a card that can be inserted in the back of most machines and is sent to you by your home care provider. The information is then sent back to the lab so the doctor can determine if the pressure needs to be adjusted. The doctor will see if a mask leak is being shown by the data or if the time the patient uses the machine nightly is not sufficient.

Many times, the patient is called in for a lab visit or acclimation to be fitted with another mask and to address other concerns concerning using the CPAP. If no leak is evident, there has been no weight loss and it shows that compliance is an issue, the doctor can then recommend an APAP test. APAP stands for AUTO TITRATING POSITIVE AIRWAY PRESSURE. What that means is that the machine will increase or decrease airway pressure as needed by the patient while the patient sleeps. Most CPAP are continuous as the name implies, so having an APAP machine helps to eliminate the dreaded in lab titration study.

The machine is either sent to you or a representative from the home care company comes to the house to set everything up. The machine will replace your own for the test's duration as designated by the doctor, which normally lasts about a week. There are no wires that need to be attached and you will use your own hose and mask. The purpose of the machine is to determine what your optimal pressure will be at the end of the study. The CPAP pressure ranges from 4.0cm H2O to 20.0cm H20. Most patients never reach the higher pressures and many do not stay at the lower pressures. The vast majority of the population seems to end up with pressures between 10.0 cm H2O to 14.0 cm H2O that is neither good or bad...it just is. So don't get overly concerned about the actual number associated with keeping you breathing all night long and be glad that the therapy works.

Once the test is completed, the data is downloaded and the doctor reviews the results. If a decrease in pressure is needed, a prescription will be written and the change will be made. Hopefully, that will resolve the issue and you will enjoy blissful sleep for many nights to come.

CHAPTER NINE

Using your equipment

Change is inevitable - except from a vending machine.

Robert C. Gallagher

One of the biggest issues that I find with my patients is that many have never been taught how to actually use their machines. Some home care companies just ship the equipment to their patients with a DVD. I am going to assume that their research has shown that the majority of these patients are able to view and understand the instructions on the DVD, set up the equipment and start using their CPAP with no issues. I am also going to assume that in the vast majority of instances, this may be true. Unfortunately, I have been confronted with many patients who have received the machine in this manner and have tried to set up their equipment and failed miserably on many levels. Other DME providers send out a representative to help the patient with the initial setup. This first contact allows the patients to ask questions, learn to put on the mask and get acquainted with using their CPAPs. Unfortunately. I have also heard from patients who at times, are seated at the kitchen table when being fitted with their mask. This does not allow the patients to experience using the mask as they would when they go to bed. Again, when the representative leaves, the patients are left to struggle trying to adjust the mask at night while the pressure slowly increases in strength or worst they inadvertently start the machine at their prescribed pressure settings and are overwhelmed with air pressure, mask and leaks

Let us touch on the sleep study one more time. The study with the masks and machine allows the tech and the doctors to determine what pressure you need when you are sleeping, that will allow you to breathe consistently all night long. In other words, your therapeutic pressure is the amount of air that is needed to keep your airway open nightly. Once that is determined, most doctors write a prescription with that pressure along with orders for a machine and all the accessories to be sent to the patient. At that point, the doctor's initial interaction is over until the follow-up visit. The doctors assume that all will go as planned once the prescription is sent to the corresponding DME provider.

Simply put, doctors expect and at times, demand that their patients use their CPAP religiously on a nightly basis. That concept is well and good in theory, but it only works if the patient's apnea is severe and they are very sleepy. For the most part, patients try to use the machine and start having issues from the onset. Remember the Autonomic Nervous System? Well, for those of you that are not into biology, I am going to throw you a curve ball. There is more to you than that. There is also the Somatic Nervous system. That is the conscious you, or to put it very simply...the awake you. That is what allows you to hold on to whatever it is that you are reading. It is the part of you that consciously slows down your breathing. It is that part that makes you take Yoga Breaths. And even though normally the two never meet, it is the interaction of the awake you and the sleeping you that forms the learning curve, or the time it takes you to get accustomed to the machine. It is the combination of both these sides of you that play a big part in getting acclimated to the machine.

I was talking to a patient recently. He is a wonderful gentleman and a professor of law at the university. He told me that he would emphasis to his students the importance of talking to their clients as if they were talking to a 12 year old or a fifth grader. I had heard that statement at some other point in my life and I found it refreshing that it was still a crucial learning technique. So what does this have to do with the two sides of you? The sleeping you is managed by, on an evolutionary level, an old part of the brain known as the brain stem. Remember that it never understands and only reacts to its environment; so, it is only through repetition that it can capture the essence of what needs to be done. In other words, no matter how you come to the realization that CPAP is going to be a vital part of your life, and no matter how committed you are to sleeping with it nightly, the autonomic nervous system may react in an entirely different manner. That is why every person reacts to using CPAP in his or her own unique way, hence the learning curve.

For some patients the learning curve is short. The brain adjusts to the constant flow of air and the patient is able to sleep throughout the night with no issues. For other patients, this time of adjustment can extend over a longer period. Issues with anxiety, claustrophobia, insomnia or learned behavior can greatly influence how a patient responds to using a CPAP machine. Other things that cause the brain difficulty in adjusting are the type of apnea that the patient actually has. For example, it is more common that women suffer from REM related OSA. When a patient has this, the events are clustered primarily when the patient is in REM. The overall average of the index, or the amount of times a person has events per hour, may be low due to the clustering. Yet if the average is isolated only when the patient is in REM sleep, that index soars. When a patient with Rem related OSA is placed on CPAP, the brain may fight the air current when the patient is in any other stage of sleep but loves that air pressure when it goes into the REM cycle. Many of my patients complain that they do not feel any different when using CPAP and it is because it is going to take time for the autonomic nervous system to realize that the pressurized air is going to be flowing all night long. The "fighting" or adjustment period is caused by the arousals that the brain is having when not in REM. The arousals can be compared to an annoyance to the brain that causes the brain to go from a deeper stage of sleep to a lighter stage of sleep to try and adjust itself to the continuous air pressure. It is, at times a long process and patience is the key. Eventually, the autonomic nervous system will realize that the constant airflow is not going away. It will adapt and work with the air in the same manner that it adapts to you being outside on a blustery day. It is what it is, nothing more and nothing less.

Mild sleep apnea can cause the same havoc with the sleeping you. There are just not enough events to cause the brain to easily accept the use of constant air pressure. Again time, patience and perseverance is the key. The idea of a PAP-NAP is gaining popularity in the sleep community. This "naps" that are conducted in the sleep centers last about three hours. The patient is fitted with a mask and then is placed on CPAP. Breathing techniques similar to the yoga breaths that I recommend are used. The patient is allowed and actually encouraged to fall asleep during this time period in the hopes that through exposure to the machine, the patient's resistance to using a CPAP is minimized. Some labs incorporate aromatherapy along with soothing music and dim lights to give the patient a sense of comfort and help in relaxation. Research has shown that these techniques increase the ease with which a patient adapts to CPAP. Can these techniques be used in the privacy of the patients' home? I am certainly of the opinion that any technique that helps a patient breathe better at night is wonderful. Remember that the goal of a CPAP is to hold the airway open during the period that a person sleeps. Sleep is needed for its restorative properties, and it is a vital part of our lives.

When setting up the CPAP in your home, try to keep the machine level to or slightly lower than your head. The nightstand is a good base or even a wooden chair works well. Some patients have told me that they have built shelves to hold the machine in place. You just want to keep in mind that the machine cannot be higher than your head so you will avoid the siphon effect especially when using humidity. You do not want to wake up with a mouthful of water. Placement of the hose is another important factor in using your CPAP. As I previously mentioned, rainout or condensation are parameters that must be considered, especially in the colder months, when using the humidifier. But, the hose itself can sometimes be a big bother. Your machine will come with a 6 ft. hose standard. There are 8 ft. hoses that are sold over the Internet or locally at your home care company. One patient of mine stuck and taped two 6 ft. hoses together to make a 12 ft.

hose to allow him more freedom of movement while he slept.

Other patients complain that the hose is too long and they are afraid that they will get tangled up with it in the bed. Some patients have used hooks that they have screwed into the wall adjacent to the bed and draped the hose over the hook so the hose attaches to the mask from above. In this way, they avoid tangling themselves with it while they sleep because the hose hangs above their head. If your bed has a headboard, it can serve the same function draping the hose in a similar fashion.

I would tend to be a bit concerned if movement in bed is sufficient to allow a patient to get tangled up in the hose. I would probably recommend that the doctors set the patient up with an auto titration study that would be performed in the comfort of their house to check the pressure settings on the patient. Weight gain or weight loss is also a reason that the pressure should be checked.

One of the most common causes of disruptive sleep over time is the cumulative problems with the masks and machines itself. Time and again, patients make appointments with me to lament the woes of their masks. Horror stories abound and frustration reigns. It is understandable to consider these patients as desperate but what truly scares me are all those people who have not set foot back into the sleep labs or even talked to the DME providers or their doctors for a very long time. These patients love their machines, use them religiously, and feel that all their sleepless nights are behind them. They continue on and on with their machines and their masks guiding the air down their throats and into their lungs. Each day begins with a clear head and a rested body. But time marches on for their machines as it does for all of nature in general, and things start to break down. It would seem logical that at this point, a phone call would be in order. Alas, for many, that doesn't happen. They continue to use their beloved CPAPs and their masks.

The worst case that I had come across was a patient who came in to see me with a mask that was taped up with duct tape. Several years had transpired since he was originally set up with his machine. The mask he brought in to the lab was the original mask given to him. This patient used his mask religiously, so much so that the efficacy of the mask had been completely obliterated. Instead of calling his DME provider for a replacement he started taping the mask together. Over time, the headgear had disintegrated to such a degree that the Velcro straps did not function at all. Duct tape covered the mask and straps, holding everything together. It wasn't until the silicon cushion became non-serviceable because it had ripped apart, that he finally walked into our lab. I asked him if his insurance covered CPAP accessories and he replied that he was not sure. He had never considered calling his insurance to find out. He had also totally forgotten what company had originally set him up with his machine. A simple phone call confirmed that he had been fully covered from the onset. For this patient, a that phone call placed years earlier would have resolved years of frustration.

Problems with the machine

Believe me when I tell you that your CPAP is

supposed to be quiet. The very first CPAP was a vacuum cleaner. What they did to help the patient sleep is that they drilled a hole in the wall of the garage and passed a hose that was attached to the outtake of the vacuum cleaner. The hose was then attached to a mask that was fitted on the patient and the patient went to sleep with the filtered, (through the bag meant to hold what is vacuumed) pressurized air from the vacuum cleaner blowing through the wall into his face. That first CPAP was not quiet. No vacuum cleaner I have come across has ever been quiet. Even though the ancestor of your CPAP was loud and bulky, please don't assume that your machine will sound the same. Our ancestors were also loud and nomadic. Heck, some of our own family members act the same way.

Back then when we were nomadic running around hunting mastodons we probably had to be loud, but many times we cringe when a family member acts outrageously. You should also cringe if your CPAP acts like the vacuum cleaner. That is not normal. The filter at the back of your CPAP is there for a reason. It is the first line of defense against foreign objects invading your motor and your lungs. If you have pets in the house, it is recommended that the filter be changed once a month. This also is true if your house attracts lots of dust. I am not asking you to become Susie homemaker and maintain a pristine environment so your CPAP can run optimally. I only ask that you keep your CPAP that way. Over the years, I have been privy to some pretty ugly looking CPAP machines. One patient came in with a CPAP that was covered in a yellow film. As I tried to wipe it clean I realized that the machine was covered in a layer of tar. The patient was a smoker. I tried to imagine where he was smoking and how small the area was where he and his machine shared space: The size of a small closet perhaps. I could not fathom how a machine could be so completely covered in a film of tar from cigarette smoke. I put on some gloves and used a commercial grade cleaner and wiped down the machine while explaining to the patient the importance of proper machine hygiene. He responded by stating that he was trying to quit. I hoped that seeing how his smoking affected he machine would further motivate him to attain his goal. Another time a patient came in with a CPAP that he had been using religiously for about 10 years. He complained that a couple of nights earlier his CPAP had stopped working. He stated that he could hear the motor running, but no air was coming out. He pulled out the machine and it was inspected. The filter was pulled out from back of the machine. It was so dirty that it was black and compressed. The patient stated that he had never realized that there was a filter that needed to be changed. TEN YEARS and not once was the filter inspected. Once the filter was removed, the machine was turned on. A puff of dust blew out of the front of the machine and the air started flowing as it was meant to flow.

This patient was well dressed, had an important job and was well respected by his colleagues. He was not a vagrant, mentally deficient or lacking in common sense. He just didn't know.

CHAPTER TEN

Masks, masks and more masks

"One day you wake up and realize the world can be conquered...
I'm going to put a mask on and scrawl my name across the face
of the world, build cities of gold, come back and stomp this place
flat, until even the bricks are just dust. So you can just shut up.
All of you... I'm going to move the world."

Austin Grossman

The hardest part about CPAP is choosing a mask that will work for you nightly without causing undue pain and discomfort. Before diving into the masks that, at the present time, seem to be the best on the market, I want to help you prepare for using the mask by giving some pointers.

 First, please make sure that your face is clean. Wash it with soap and water and nothing else. That means no creams, no over the counter lotions, nothing that can cause a slick surface for the mask to slide on. If your face tends to be oily, make sure that you use some type of astringent to help close the pores. Cold water also works well for this purpose.

Second, make sure that all the parts of the mask are assembled correctly. If you put the mask on, tighten it and still experience a lot of whistling, hissing or some other type of noise, please check to make sure that it was put back together properly.

Third, don't be afraid to try different masks. The mask that you used in the sleep lab does not have to be the one that you have to stick with forever. Try several masks till you find one that is comfortable. Remember, new masks are being developed regularly. I have listed a variety of masks, some older models and some newer, that work for the majority of CPAP users. The big four CPAP manufacturers are represented, along with some other companies in no particular order, so hopefully you will be able to find a good fit. Before we delve into the different types of masks available on the market, the following should be stated...

A word of caution about any mask containing any type of blue gel.

Though the manufacturers state that all the parts of the masks are hypoallergenic, there are cases where patients develop an allergic reaction to the chemical component used in the making of the gel. Reactions include skin breakdown, sneezing. or cold-like symptoms. If this happens to you, please do not worry needlessly. Just call your DME provider to be fitted with a silicone mask instead.

NASAL PILLOWS

AN IMPORTANT NOTE WHEN USING NASAL PILLOWS.

Be careful to make sure that when you bring the mask to the face you can see the opening of the pillows forming an upside down "**V**". IF THE PILLOWS ARE NOT PLACED IN THE HEADGEAR CORRECTLY, THERE WILL BE INCREASED DISCOMFORT, IRRITATION AND PAIN.

The following nasal pillows are listed in no specific order.

ResMed Swift II Nasal Pillows

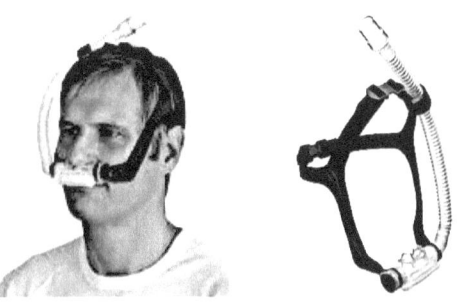

The first of the Swift series of nasal pillow. It has a side attached hose that can be changed from one side to the other. A good mask for side sleepers... The headgear has an upper band that sits on the top of the head like a headband and a bottom strap that sits at the area up and down till the pillows are in the nostrils and are completely blocking any air from escaping. When the mask in on properly, there should be no hissing, except for the air that escapes the exhalation port in the front of the mask. To secure the mask to the face, first tighten the upper band till the side of the mask is resting above the ears in the same place the arms of your glasses would be. Tighten the back band to secure in place. Last, swivel the cushion. The hose can be switched from one side to the other by pulling out the hose on one end and pulling out the plug on the other end and reversing them.

ResMed Swift LT

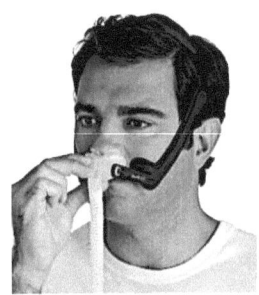 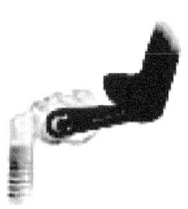

The Swift LT has the same headgear as the Swift II but the pillows are now more centered on the face. The hose is now situated in the middle of the mask. The Resmed Swift LT pillows also swivel to adjust them properly in the nostrils. Place the headgear in the same manner that you would with the Swift II. The top strap will rest at the top of the head where a headband would sit. The back band rests at the top of the neck or the base of the head. Sizes are Small, Medium, and Large.

ResMed Swift LT for her

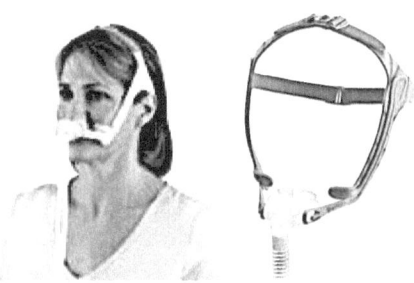

In the Swift LT version for women called the LT for her, the space between the top strap and the bottom strap is wider to allow women to pass the hair between them comfortably. The pillows range from large to extra small for petite noses. The headgear is a light blue instead of the dark blue but the mask is put on the face in the same manner.

Mirage Swift FX

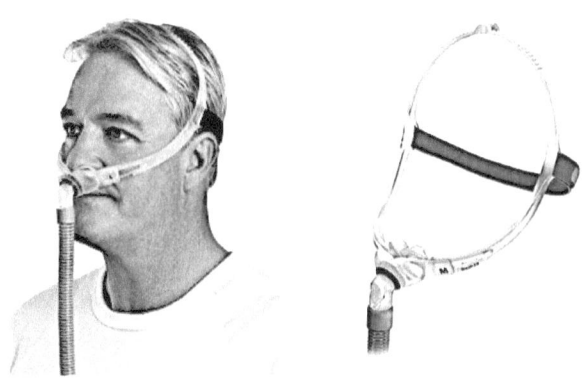

The Swift FX a nasal pillow from ResMed. The mask is made totally from silicone with a small adjustable band that sits at the base of the skull. The top piece has teeth that help to adjust the mask upwards. Again, only tighten the top portion of the mask until it sits approximately in the same place that your glasses would rest over your ears. This pillow system does not swivel so it is important that you tighten the mask to your face by tightening the band that hugs the base of the skull on the back of the neck. There is also the FX for her. Sizes range from large to extra small.

Swift Bella FX

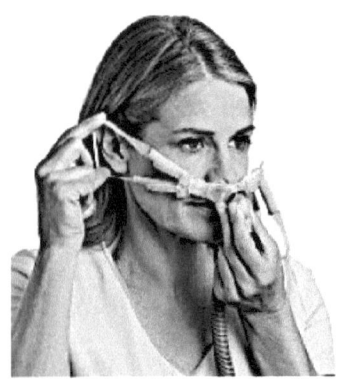

ResMed has introduced new headgear specifically designed to be used by women. The mask is the standard FX pillow design but the headgear anchors around the ears to hold the mask securely in place. The complaint of many women who have to use CPAP is that the straps used to hold the mask in place ruin their hairdos. This mask resolves that basic issue.

Respironics GoLife Nasal Pillows

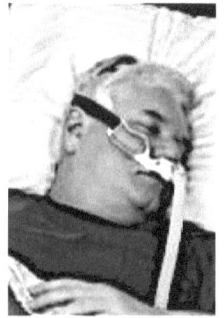 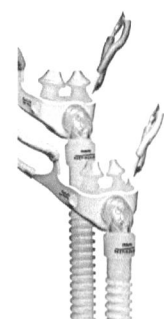

This is another nasal pillow on the market with a 360-degree swivel, and anchors that mold to the specific contours of the male or female face. The headgear has straps on either side and on the top to adjust the pillows to reduce leaks and aid in comfort. The pillow sizes range from petite to large to accommodate most patients' needs.

Fisher Paykel Opus Nasal Pillows

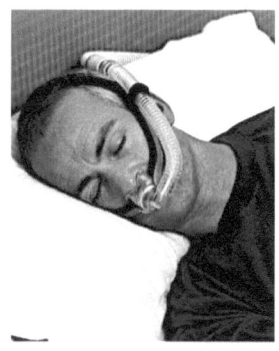 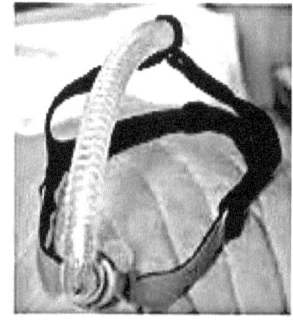

A simple nasal pillow with few parts that also allows the

patient to sleep in any position. There are adjustments at the top and on the back of the headgear to adjust the mask to fit securely on the face. It also has a Velcro ring that allows the patient to shift the hose to the side or to the top of the head for those who sleep on their stomach or sides

Fisher Paykel Pilairo nasal pillows

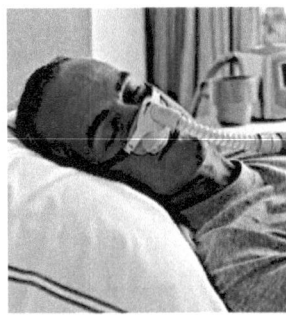 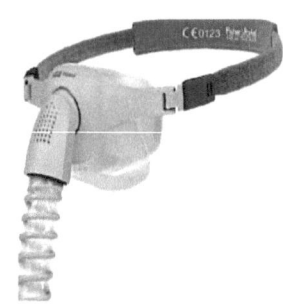

The Pilairo nasal pillows are the newest mask design for use with CPAP. Light, visual unobtrusive and equipped with only one strap, the Pilairo is comfortable and easy to use. It was designed with three components...the strap, the pillow and the hose. The minimal design of the mask makes it easy to clean. The pillows inflate with air and surround the nostrils forming a seal while delivering the needed pressure. The strap is auto-adjusting to fit most patients. The hose, as in all pillow designs, attaches to the CPAP hose with ease.

Respironics Nuance and Nuance Pro

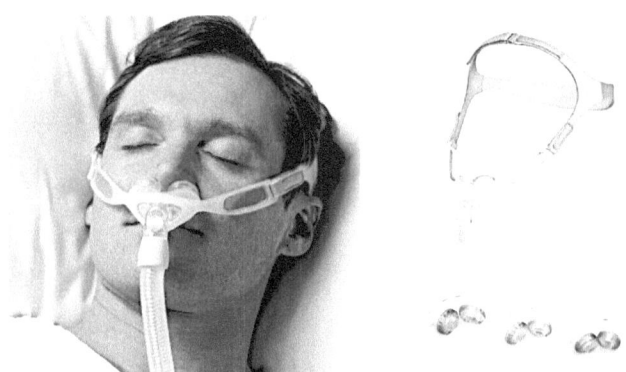

The first gel nasal pillows on the market; the pillows come in three sizes...small, medium and large, to fit a wide range of different size nostrils. The headpiece has a choice of a gel or fabric frame that helps reduce those annoying red marks that may appear on the face after using a mask overnight. The back of the headgear seems to sit higher on the head and may cause some instability, especially with longer hair on women. That may be one of the few drawbacks. Make sure the top piece of the head gear sits on the top of the head or a little farther back to allow the bottom section of the headgear to sit closer to the nape of the neck for increased stability. The top strap should also be adjusted, if needed, for added stability and comfort.

ResMed AirFit P10

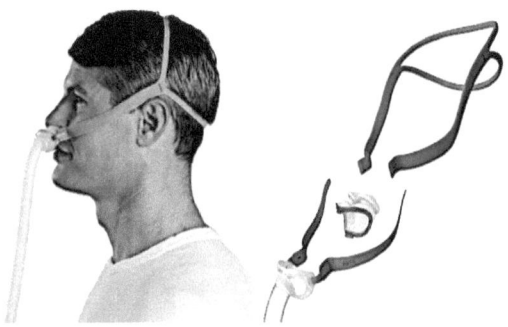

ResMed states that this mask is 50% quieter due to the newly designed woven mesh air venting and 50% lighter than the ever-popular Swift masks. It has three pieces that allows for easier reassembly after washing the mask. and three pillow sizes (S,M,L). The headgear splits in a Y shape allowing the mask to be anchored on the top and back of the head. As with many ResMed masks, there is a version for her.

Puritan Bennett Breeze nasal pillows

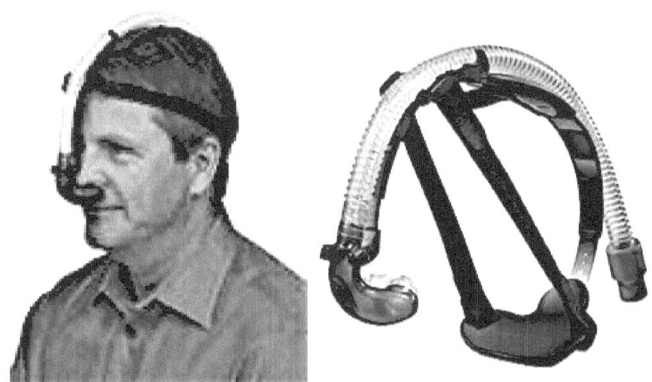

The Puritan Bennett Breeze mask is ideal for patients who prefer not to have anything on their face or around the neck area. It is perfect for patients who have suffered neck injuries or have any issues concerning the neck area. It is also recommended for people who sleep on their stomachs. The mask has a hard plastic piece that rests on the back of the head. It is anchored by two straps on either side that provide lateral support and attach to the front and back of the headgear. The straps are adjustable bay tightening or loosening the Velcro straps. The pillows, which come in small, medium, and large sizes, can also be adjusted for a more comfortable fit by adjusting inward or outward till the pillows fit securely in the nostrils. The plastic plate sits at the base of the head and the metal support that rests on the top of the head can also be adjusted by sliding the curved bar inward or outward to fit the patient snugly.. This design allows no pressure to be placed on the neck providing less tension to areas of the neck that may be compromised. The front of the mask is adjustable, angling in towards the nose or outwards and can be moved to fit the nostrils comfortably.

NASAL MASKS

For many, nasal pillows have helped CPAP users sleep well throughout the night due to the minimal invasiveness of the masks. For others, the force of the air can irritate the inner lining of the nose causing pain, a burning sensation and even nose bleeds. This is where a nasal mask can make a difference. Though the difference in the flow of the air into the nasal passages is delayed by milliseconds; (because the air comes up the hose, bounces off the face and back into the mask causing turbulence from which the patient breathes the pressurized air) the brain immediately registers it. Those milliseconds can mean all the difference in the world for a patient who cannot tolerate nasal pillows. It can also be the difference between being compliant with the machine or total non-compliance. Again, the masks are listed in no specific order.

Fisher Paykel Eson Nasal mask

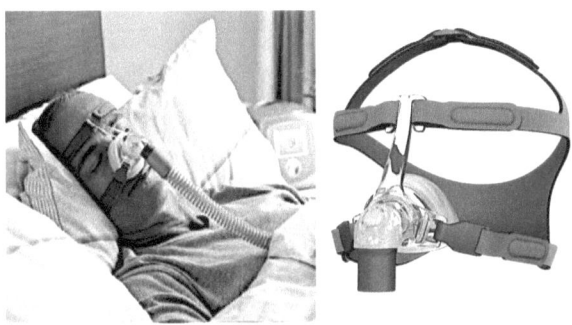

The Eson is a new nasal mask that features the roll fit seal. This allows the mas to "roll" back and forth on the bridge of the nose to form a comfortable seal. The Eson also features Velcro straps with Easy clip hooks that allows the mask to be easily secured to the face: This is done by pushing the hook into the vertical bar on the mask. Removal is just as easy with a simple twisting motion to unhook the clip from the bar. The type of feature works for patients that suffer from arthritis and have difficulty with hand dexterity or fine hand movements. The mask also has a Velcro strap on the top of the headgear to further adjust the mask up or down on the nose and aids in stabilizing the mask on the face. The frame is designed to accept small, medium or large interfaces and the bar that attaches to the forehead straps are narrow enough to allow for a clear line of vision. The ball and socket elbow where the hose attaches to the mask rotates more freely allowing for less drag from the hose.

Respironics Wisp Nasal Mask

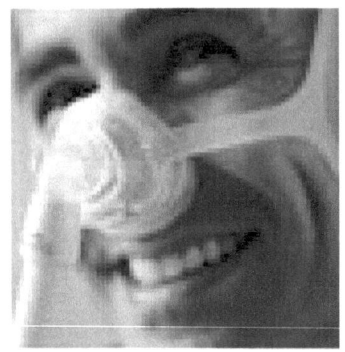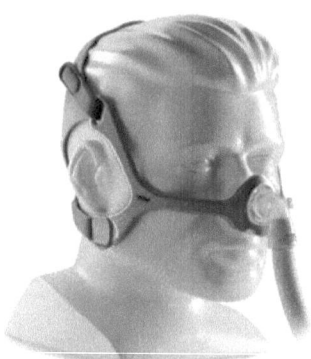

This is another new mask to be developed for CPAP users. It offers the same visual unobtrusive feature of the nasal pillows with the comfort of the nasal mask. Unlike the nasal pillows that sit in the nostrils, the Wisp covers sit on the nose like the traditional nasal mask but are significantly smaller. It has a small triangular interface but it lacks the vertical bar that connects to the forehead piece. This allows a patient to read or watch television and use his or her glasses if needed   It is anchored to the head by a head piece that rests on the top of the head and around the neck. It comes with Velcro straps to adjust tightness. The other major difference with this mask is that it can be supplied with a silicone headgear that holds the mask or a cloth headgear. Clinical trials have shown that patients prefer the silicone while home care companies prefer the cloth. The cloth is also reversible with a smooth side that can rest on the face or a cushier side for overall comfort.

Fisher Paykel Zest Nasal Mask

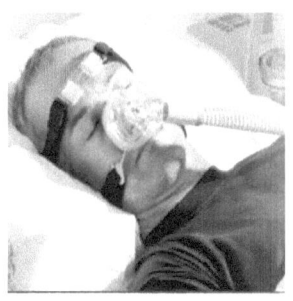 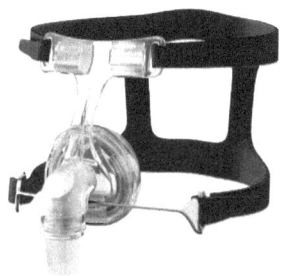

The Zest is also a simple mask with few parts. The translucent white cover sits over the gray foam that fits in the channel in the hard plastic. The wide foam allows for a good seal with very few removable parts. It is offered in a petite, standard and wide size. The slight curve on the clear plastic that connects to the forehead allows the mask to sit slightly angled off the bridge of the nose thus reducing pressure and preventing irritation to that sensitive area. There have been some patients who do have an allergic reaction to the grey foam. If that occurs, a mask with an all-silicone interface is the only other alternative. The headgear has a pliable bar that sits in a channel on the mask near the exhalation port. It is meant to slide from side to side to help to maintain the seal on the face if the patient shifts during the night. This bar also is designed with a hook to simplify the removal of the mask in the morning without having to undo the Velcro strap.

ResMed Mirage FX Nasal Mask

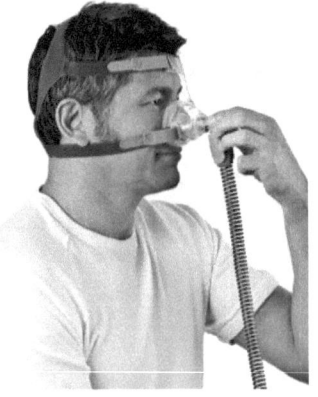 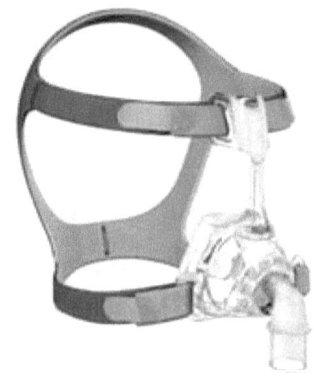

One of the newest masks on the market, it is very light and user friendly. It has a butterfly hinge on the forehead that reduces pressure marks. The wings spread apart as the straps are tightened or loosened when the headgear is adjusted to prevent leaks. The back section of the mask where the exhalation port is located, has a soft clip that can be pressed and separated from the interface if the patient needs to disconnect from the CPAP without taking off the mask. This clip stays connected to the hose and can easily be snapped back in when the patient returns to the bed.

The mask also comes in a version for her with a pink headgear to make it more attractive to female patients.

Sleepweaver Nasal Cloth Mask

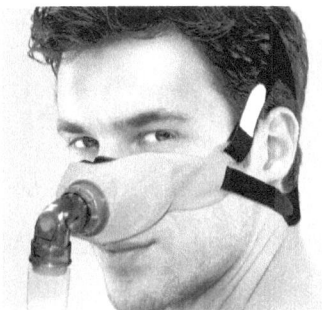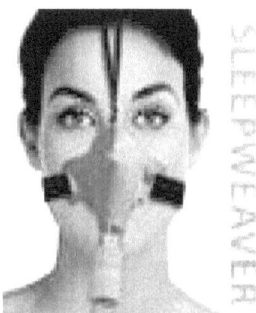

The only cloth mask on the market: One size fits all so it may not be good for wide noses or very petite noses. It is visually unobtrusive and the band that goes up between the eyes is so narrow that glasses can be worn with it. It is also the only mask that can be washed in the washing machine. The material comes in a variety of colors and prints. It inflates like a balloon providing a good seal and a comfortable fit. The major issue that some patients have mentioned with this mask is that the plastic piece that attaches to the hose rests on the upper lip under the nose and may be somewhat bothersome. It primarily works well at low air pressure settings.

The mask is also offered in a variety of prints that available along with the solid colors shown above.

ResMed AirFit

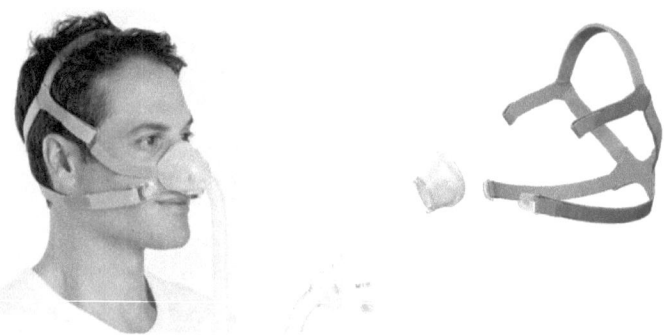

One of the unique benefits of this mask are the magnetic tabs that audibly click on the front and attach the headgear to the mask. This mask is wonderful for people with arthritis since no snapping or clipping is involved. Once the headgear is adjusted to fit the patient the magnetic clips do the rest. Some redness on the bridge of the nose may occur due to how the mask rests on the face. This can be remedied by adjusting the angle of the mask on the bridge of the nose. As always, make sure the seal is intact and no leaks occur.

ResMed Soft Gel Nasal Mask

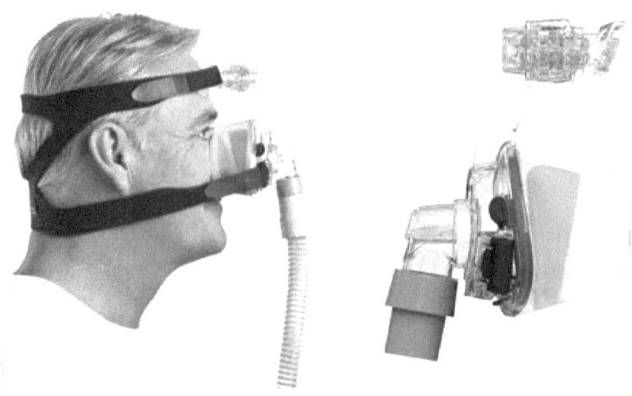

This is a heavier mask. It has a thick blue silicone gel that transitions to a less dense clear gel. Very cushy if the weight is not a bother. Very good seal. The headgear is tightened in the same manner as any other nasal mask with Velcro straps at the top and clips at the bottom.

This mask also has a knob on the "T" portion of the mask that allows 24 micro adjustments to the angle of the mask against the face. It can be turned to the right to angle the mask away from the bridge of the nose and to the left to bring it closer. This helps in controlling leaks near the eyes.

Respironics Comfort Gel Blue Nasal Mask

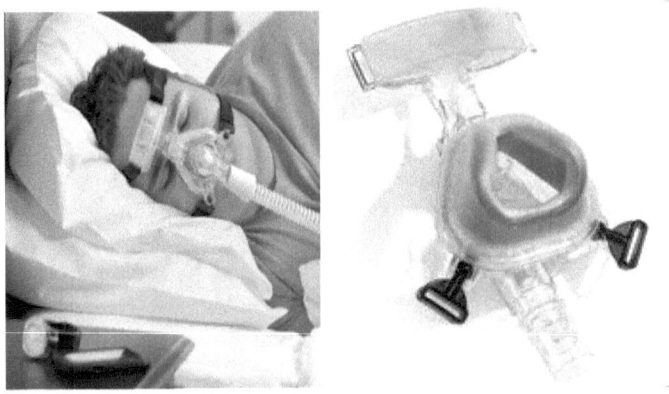

Nice starter mask with a translucent white cover and an inner blue gel cushion. This is a favorite of many sleep labs to run overnight titrations on patients. The blue gel defuses the pressure when the mask is tightened to the face to insure a good seal. It has a few more parts and it is important to return the blue seal with the cover to the hard plastic once the mask has been pulled apart for cleaning. The anchors have rounded heads so that the headgear can be hooked into the slots at the base of the mask. It was also designed to allow it to be turned or flipped up within the socket to help to shorten the headgear for those people who have smaller heads. To clarify, just imagine rolling something up to shorten the length. That is the other feature of this mask.

Respironics Easylife Nasal Mask

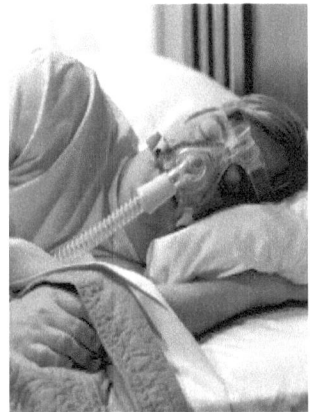 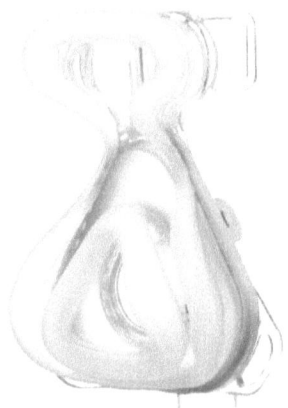

This is another self-sealing nasal mask. The patented auto seal technology allows the user to place the mask on the face and turn on the CPAP allowing the air pressure to seal the mask to the nose. The main support for this mask rests on the forehead straps. The straps that go around the neck are kept fairly loose so the air in the mask can be used to inflate and seal the mask against the skin. The bottom straps should only be tightened enough to stop any hissing or leaking where the mask rests against the face. This is a light mask putting very little pressure on the face. Cleaning may be a little difficult for elderly or handicapped patients due to the inner and outer interface associated with the mask, as can be seen in the photograph, especially when the mask has to be reassembled. The availability of mask sizes ranges from small to extra large along with a wide interface. The headgear has straps that can be adjusted to give further stability to the mask. It also has a clip that attaches to the mask to allow increased ease of use.

Resmed Mirage Activa Nasal

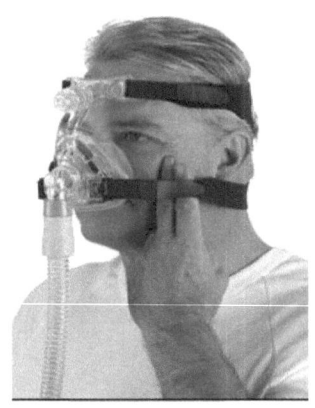 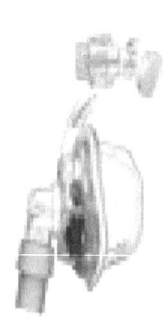

This mask is good for people who want the comfort of a nasal mask but like to sleep on their sides. This mask "inflates" like a balloon when placed on the face and the air from the CPAP is flowing. This mask should be held securely on the forehead similar to the way that Pocahontas wore her headband around her head. The lower strap should sit loosely and be tightened only enough to prevent air leaks. The part of the mask touching the nose will "float" moving to either side

as a person shifts from one side to the other. Notice how the model has two fingers placed between the face and the strap. This is done to make sure that the strap I loose enough to allow the interface to inflate properly.

There is a blue ring that sits inside a groove in the clear silicone. Once inserted properly, the blue wings on either side of the mask will clip into the hard outer plastic shell.

FULL FACE MASKS

The full face mask is normally the first mask that a sleep tech will use on the patient. The reasoning for this stems from that fact that many people who suffer from sleep apnea tend to be mouth breathers. This type of mask allows the patient to breathe through the mouth or nose without losing the benefit of the air. As mentioned in a previous chapter, many patients who were considered mouth breathers when starting CPAP, may not be so once the brain retrains itself to breathe exclusively through the nose. Some hints to take into consideration is the fact that even though a patient is using a full face mask, the machine is run without any humidity and the patient wakes up without suffering from a dry mouth. If this happens to you, try to switch to a nasal mask or a nasal pillow. For obvious reasons, it may be a better fit.

The following full face masks are presented in no specific order...

Resmed Quattro FX Full Face Mask

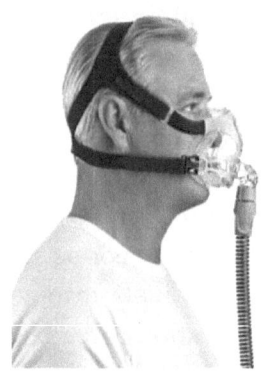 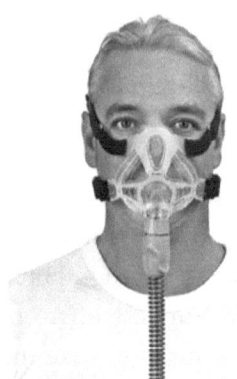

Think of this mask as another full face that allows a patient to wear glasses to read or watch television while having the mask on the face. The cushion should rest about halfway down the bridge of the nose. The bottom of the mask will then rest about a half inch beneath the lower lip. A good way to verify that the mask is positioned correctly is by resting a pair of glasses on the bridge of the nose. If the glasses rest comfortably and are not riding up on the face, then the mask is correctly placed on the face. If the glasses ride up, then bring the mask down farther by adjusting and tightening the lower straps. This will bring the mask down further on the nose and anchor it on the face correctly. This mask runs larger than normal, so make sure that you are fitted with a size smaller than what you are accustomed to using.

To tighten the mask, it is important to remember to tighten the lower straps first. This will pull the mask down farther on the face to improve the seal. Using the upper straps to tighten the mask will cause the lateral curls seen inside the seal to ride up causing a leak near the eyes. As in all Resmed masks, there are clips that will release the mask when pinched. One of the biggest concerns with this mask is that in some patients, it tends to rid up the nose during the night. The only way this may be prevented is, as previously stated, by tightening the lower strap more to keep the mask sitting lower on the bridge of the nose.

Fisher Paykel Forma Full Face mask

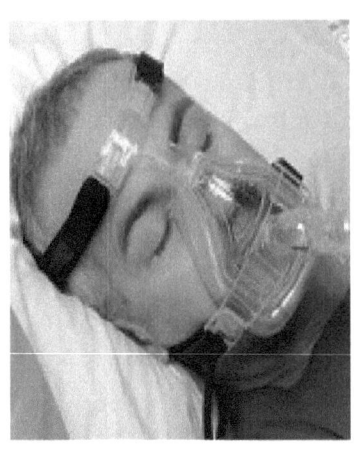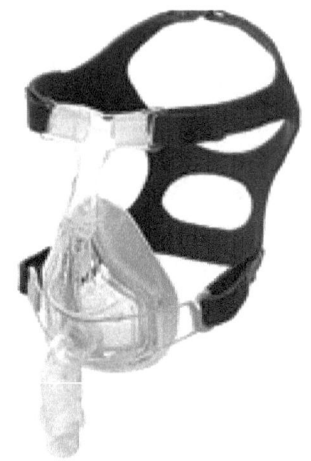

The Forma has a feature that is unique to full face masks. It's like having two masks in one. It can be used with or without the foam insert. It is also one of two masks on the market that currently sits under the chin to aid in preventing the mouth from dropping open. The grey foam gives the mask more substance that may increase comfort of the mask for some patients. The foam insert and the translucent outer cover sit inside the channels or grooves found on the hard plastic face piece. The mask has two hooks that allow the headgear to be removed without compromising the fit on the patient. Since the placement of this mask starts under the chin, it is very important that the mask lean out away from the face when fitting it. The two straps that are used to adjust the mask are the bottom straps first and then the straps at the top of the head. The forehead straps rarely come into play when adjusting for a good fit.

ResMed AirFit F10

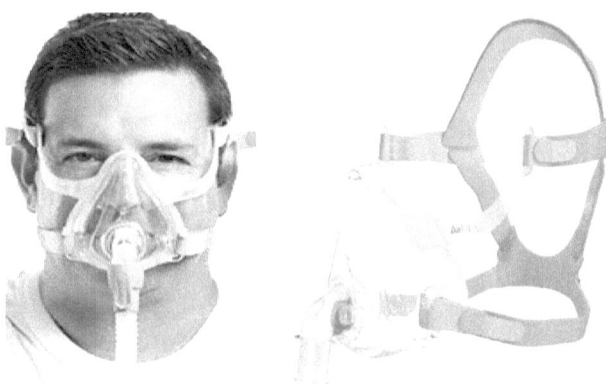

The AirFit F10 is the lightest of the ResMed full face product line. It is composed of four parts making it easier to assemble than most of the full face masks on the market. It was designed with circular defused venting that allows the air to leave the mask port without bothering the patient's bed partner. It may be difficult for patients with arthritis because there is still strap adjustment necessary to maintain a good seal. Like the Quattro FX, there is no upper support allowing a clear line of vision so the patient can read or watch TV comfortably.

Respironics Amara Full Face mask

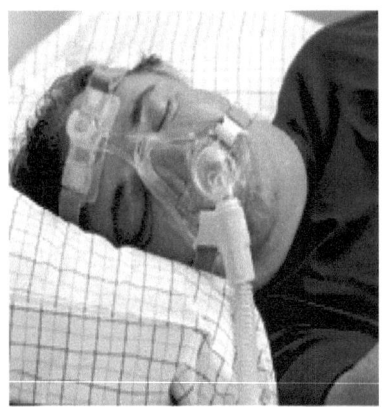 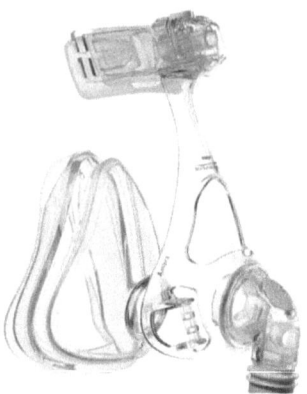

This is one of the newest full face masks on the market. It combines many winning features of previous masks along with a new design to give a lighter, easy to assemble mask that fits the vast majority of CPAP users who prefer having a full face mask. It offers a one-click technology allowing the patient to change the size of the interface or replace worn interfaces with new ones by clicking them into place. To remove the cushion, just pull to release it from the frame. A large circular hole is found in each cushion with a clear plastic ring. Take the new cushion and push it into the frame till it clicks in place. The mask is now ready to be worn. The frame is designed to accept all sizes, minimizing the complexity of upkeep. It also has a very simple attachment for affix the headgear to the mask. It clips in by pushing the "C" shaped clasp into the bar on the frame. To remove the mask, simply twist the clasp and it will release from the bar. The forehead can be adjusted by moving the slider at the top of the mask inward or outward.

Respironics Comfort Gel Full Face mask

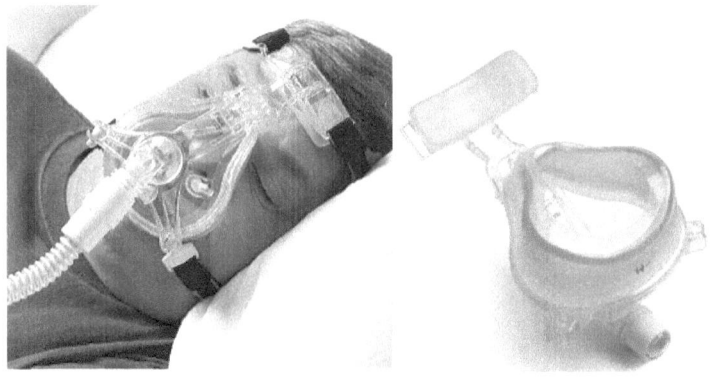

This mask was designed based on the popularity of the comfort gel nasal mask, but instead if just covering the nose, it covers the nose and mouth. It has the same features as the nasal version. It is made up of a blue gel inner portion that is covered by a translucent white interface. It has an adjustable forehead setting with a hinge that can be moved to four different angles by pressing on the clip and releasing the hinge. This allows the mask to be brought in closer or farther away from the nose to adjust for leaks. It also has ball joints to allow for pivoting of the bottom strap of the headgear to make it smaller. In this way it can be adjusted to fit smaller heads. One other feature of this mask is that there is a small port on the mask itself that can be opened to connect an oxygen hose to the mask is the patient needs to have oxygen delivered while on CPAP. It is important that this vent is always closed when using the machine at night. If it is open air will escape and the therapeutic pressure needed to keep the airway open will be reduced.

ResMed Quattro Full Face Mask

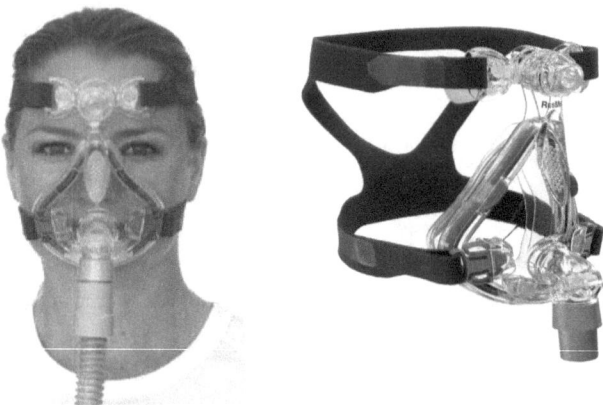

This is a non-gel Full face mask that has a clear knob that can be rotated to micro adjust mask closer to or farther away from the nose. The mask comes in three sizes...small, medium, and large. There is a "T" or the portion that rests on the forehead. It is connected to the nasal portion by a clip. This clip adjusts the angle of the mask by pushing the mask more tightly to the bridge of the nose or moving it away. It functions like the claws on a crab. Pinching them together loosens the "T" and allows the mask to move in or out.\

All three sizes have a good portion of the silicon covering that rests on the face actually putting lots of pressure on the nose, not very good for people who have high nose bridges because it tends to cause soreness or blistering over time. So if you have a Roman nose, this is not the mask for you. There is also a channel where a blue ring has to be inserted. It is important that this ring is inserted correctly or else leaks can occur.

This is also not a mask that is good for elderly patients because of the number of parts that make up the mask as shown below unless there is a caregiver who can work with the patient and the mask.

Mirage Liberty Full Face Mask

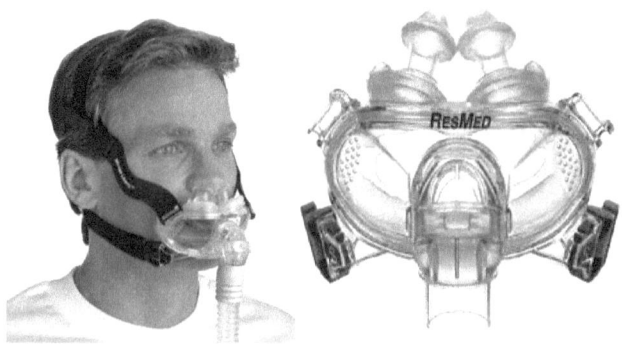

This is a combination mask. It incorporates the pillows but also has a piece that covers the mouth. It is a mask that may work for patients who want a full face mask but do not want something that is visually intrusive. Glasses can be worn with this mask that would allow reading or watching TV. One of the complaints that I have had with this mask is that some patients complain of excessive air pressure from the pillows.

The pillows come in three sizes...large to small, as does the mouth piece. The pillows are also independent of each other so if one nostril is larger than the other, two different size pillows can be inserted to improve fit. *This mask HAS to be placed on the face, pillows first.* Anchor the pillows in the nose then drop the rest of the mask over the mouth. The top straps adjust the angle of the pillows to aid in sealing the nostrils and the bottom straps tighten the mask over the mouth to prevent leaks. If placed properly, it is a good mask for mouth breathers. The bottom straps have clips that if squeezed, will separate the mask from the headgear for easy removal.

Respcare Hybrid Full face mask

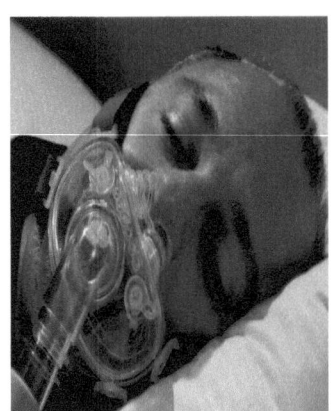 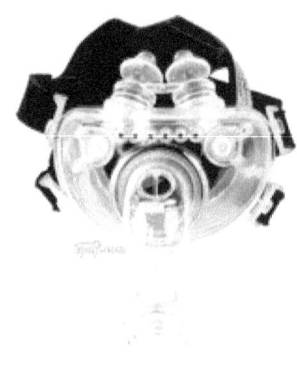

Another full face/nasal pillow mix that is similar to the Resmed Liberty. The pillow sizes can also be adjusted depending on the size of the nasal opening. Each pillow can also be changed independently to adapt to the individual's nose. The lower part comes in small, medium, and large to fit each patient uniquely. It is a mask that also allows patients to read or watch television without the cumbersome "T" that many of the other full face masks have for added support on the forehead. The straps clip onto the mask, which can be difficult for patients who have problems with manual dexterity or fine muscle movement.

Fisher Paykel Oracle mouth mask

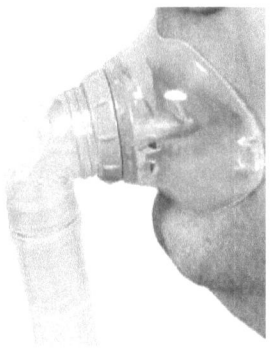 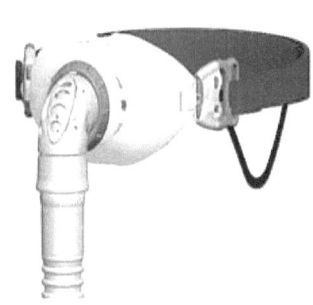

The only mouth mask on the market, good for patients who have use of only one side of their bodies (ie., stroke patients) or only one hand available to adjust the mask. Initially, extensive drooling may occur and nasal plugs also accompany the mask so no nasal breathing occurs. These issues resolve themselves after about two weeks. The mask has two portions, one that sits inside the mouth in front of the teeth and an outer portion that covers the lips. The large ring is used to compress the inner and outer portions so that the lips are sandwiched between them. This keeps the mask in place and prevents leaks. It also has an optional band that can be wrapped around the head for added support against leak.

For patients new to the mask, one of the biggest problems that occur is that there is an increased amount of saliva formed by the body when the mask is in place. It takes the body about one week to learn to breathe with the mask and at that point the production of saliva will return to normal.

CHAPTER ELEVEN

CPAP machines, what is best for you

Harvard Law: Under the most rigorously controlled conditions of pressure, temperature, humidity, and other variables, the organism will do as it damn well pleases.

Anonymous

There is a large assortment of CPAP machines available on the market. Over the years, I have come to realize that it is better to demand a higher end machine from your DME provider than to allow them to choose the machine for you. For those of you who are not aware of how insurance works, let me explain this much. There is a standard reimbursement rate that is agreed to and followed by the varied insurance agencies in combination with the DME companies. The goal of the DME Company is to make money. Yes ultimately, they are bound to help the patient/customer, but rest assured, that if they can get away with giving patients a stripped down CPAP model, they will. That translates into more money in their pocket. This normally does not affect most CPAP users since the ultimate goal of all involved is that the patient constantly using the machine (otherwise know as CPAP compliance), and for the vast majority of patients, they will use whatever the doctor orders. As we all are aware, money makes the world go round and far be it for me to get on a soap box and say otherwise, but I only mention this because I have had the issue come up with patients who fall outside of the statistical bell curve for CPAP users. If you are one of those lucky people who will end up loving your CPAP, a basic model is fine, but there are always exceptions to that rule...and woe to those that fall into that category.

The most basic models used to deliver straight pressure. There were no extras and for those long time CPAP users, this was normally the best option for them. These users had learned to use their machines at a constant pressure, many even without the added benefit of humidity, heated or otherwise. The learning curve, or the amount of time it took for the body to adjust to CPAP, was significantly longer, but they eventually adapted. I have had patients come to me having used the CPAP with no humidity whatsoever for years. For me to add any extra options, at times, can cause more discomfort than anything else. But for patients new to the experience of using CPAP, having any and all extras helps to lessen the initial discomfort of the learning curve that exists with being trained to use the machine. I am including a varied number of machines which all perform the same functions.

The biggest concern, then, is deciding what CPAP machine is the best fit for you. The three biggest names in CPAP are Phillips Respironics, ResMed and Fisher Paykel followed by Puritan Bennett. All manufacturers offer quality machines with a two-year warranty. ResMed, Phillips Respironics and Puritan Bennett offer airflow reduction upon exhaling. They are called EPR, Flex mode and FloSense technology, respectively. These technologies allow the patient to breathe in and out with less effort; so the sense that one is fighting the airflow is minimized because the pressure increases and decreases in time with each breath.

The Fisher Paykel CPAP machine has Sensawake in the auto PAP mode. It reduces the air pressure given to the patient if the patient starts to wake up. Once the patient falls back to sleep, the machine slowly increases the air pressure to maintain the airway open.

All CPAP machines also have ramping features. This allows the air pressure to start out at a lower level and slowly increase, or ramp up, to the prescribed pressure over time. The length of time for the air pressure to reach the optimal level can range from zero to forty-five minutes and can be adjusted by the patient.

Fisher Paykel, ResMed and now Respironics, have heated tubing. This is especially beneficial for patients in colder climates. The heated tubing allows the water vapor to stay suspended as it flows up the hose while simultaneously warming the air traveling up to the patient. This reduces the uncomfortable sensation of breathing frigid air through the mask. The Fisher Paykel CPAP also offers a humidity boost mode that can provide added moisture for the patient, if needed. For those patients who have a Respironics or Puritan Bennett CPAP, hose socks are available through your home care provider. These "socks" will help to insulate the hose so the warm air can travel up the hose without condensation or "rainout" occurring. If you are feeling especially creative, or you have the ability to sew or you know someone who can do so; buy an inexpensive remnant of fleece and sew a tube. Slide the hose through and secure with rubber bands.

All CPAP machine are normally sold with a heated humidifier. Most of these units cannot be washed well and should be replaced by the DME Company from once every month to once every year. The insurance companies normally pay for these types of supplies. If you are not sure if it is covered your DME provider, call them and they should be able to tell you or simply call your insurance company and ask them directly.

All of the machines can be looked up on the Internet. Following is a list of the brands of CPAP/APAP machines currently on the market. They are listed in no particular order.

ResMed has several types of CPAP machines on the market. They are the Tango, the S8, and the newest is the S9.

ResMed S9 Series

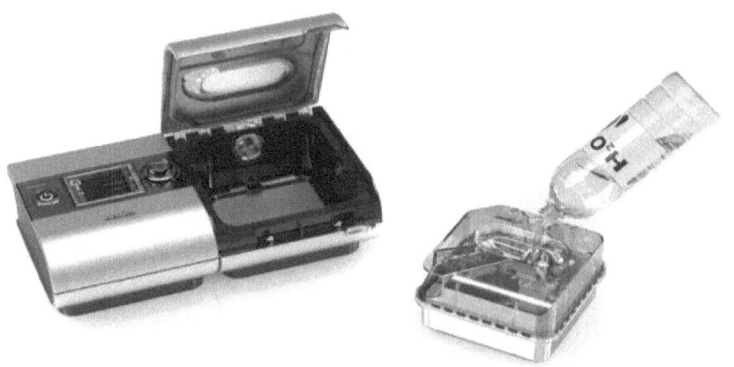

The S9 has a sleek design and you have the ability to buy skins for your PAP that can reflect your favorite team, alma mater, or print. It is the size of a shoebox with a humidifier on the right and the CPAP on the left. This machine has a color screen. The on/off button is on the left and the knob that controls all other functions is on the right. . It has a ramp feature that allows the air pressure to gradually increase over a minimum of 5 minutes to a maximum of 45 minutes to allow you to fall asleep comfortably. The starting pressure on the ramp is normally set at 4 to 6cm of water pressure. This feature is good when starting on CPAP. Once you are accustomed to using it, you may opt out of using the ramp and instead start at the prescribed pressure when going to sleep. If the ramp function is enabled, it is automatic and is normally set by the DME provider. The humidifier now can be fitted with a cleanable water chamber that can be taken apart and washed.

The CPAP itself, offers an EPR function (expiratory pressure relief) that causes the air pressure to decrease with each exhale and increase with each inhale. This ebbing and flowing of the air offers added comfort while sleeping and reduces the feel of "fighting the air" with each breath

The S9 can also be equipped with a heated hose that can help to maintain much needed moisture during the winter months. It is normally something that has to be requested. The homecare companies commonly deliver a regular hose with the unit. The heated tube is connected to the CPAP by pushing the end with the orange square into the back of the CPAP. You will then have to twist or rotate the orange fitting on the hose to fit into the orange port at the back of the machine. This will connect the copper tubing to the electricity in the CPAP. If you are provided a heated tube, the temperature inside the hose can be adjusted by tuning right knob on the right side of the color screen till the thermostat is highlighted in a darker blue on the left side of the color screen. Press the knob to turn the screen to yellow/orange and then turn the knob to the right to change the degrees setting just like the readings of a regular thermometer. Once the setting is changed, press the right knob down again to change the screen back to blue. This will set the change. The default setting is 80 degrees.

Highlighting the water droplet can also change the humidity level on the CPAP. Follow the same steps to change the heat level under the water chamber from 0 – 6 with 6 being the highest level. This controls the temperature of the hotplate under the water chamber. The EPR mode can be set with a range from 1 to 3 to maximize patient comfort.

ResMed S8

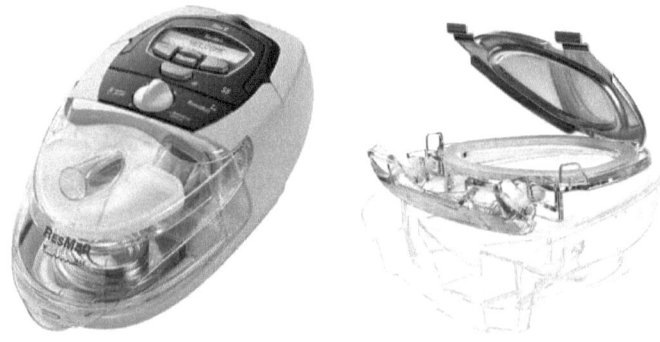

The S8 model is cream and blue and egg shaped with a clear water chamber that attaches to the front of the machine. It also has most of the features of the S9 except that it does not have a heated tube attachment. The biggest complaint of this machine was the inability to clean the water chamber well. That issue has been addressed by the production of a cleanable water chamber that allows all the nooks and crannies to be washed properly. Note though, that currently, the cleanable water chamber does not come standard with the machine and needs to be ordered separately. There may be an additional cost, but the added expense is well worth the feeling of knowing that the water chamber is free of mold and is accompanying spores.

Respironics System One Series

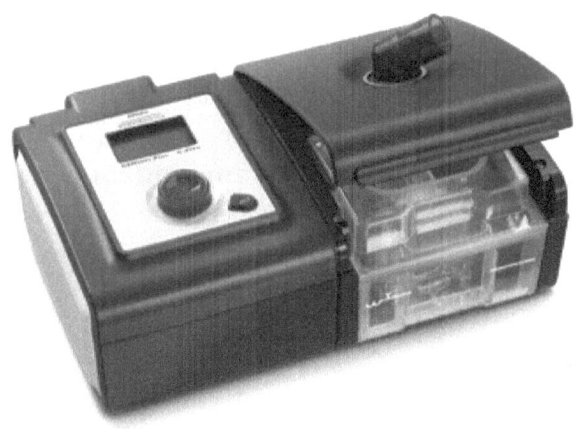

The CPAP is on the left and the humidifier is on the right. Pressing down on the knob turns on the machine. It is a very user-friendly machine with a black and white screen with four panes. The two most important panes are the Therapy screen and the flex screen. The machine will not start without having the therapy pane highlighted in the darker grey color. The Flex pane allows patients to regulate the pressure relief on the machine. The range for the pressure relief varies from 1 to 3. One is the narrowest rang, meaning that the air will back off slightly when a person exhales while using the CPAP. The 3 is the widest range. I have found, over the years, that the range of 2 seems to be the range closest to a person's normal respiratory rate. The range of 3 works best for patients that are very pressure sensitive.. This function on the machine normally has to be activated by the DME provider. If you feel the need to try it, please don't hesitate and you're your home care provider to have the Flex mode turned on.

The same knob that turns on the CPAP is also the one that regulates the humidity levels. Turning the knob to the right increases the moisture by increasing the hot plate that heats the water in the humidifier. The heat levels are from 0 to 6. **If you press down on the knob and hold it for about 10 seconds, the heater will turn on and start warming the water without running the air compressor that provides the air.** When you want to start the machine, just turn it on as usual. This feature is highly useful, especially in colder climates.

The machine also offers three modes of delivery for the humidification; the classic mode, the system one mode and the heated tube. With the humidifier set in the classic mode, only the hot plate is activated. It will heat the water and send it up the tube in the traditional manner of old. The amount of humidity will fluctuate depending on the relative humidity of the air, temperature and changes in altitude. In colder weather, this may cause the gurgling in the hose or otherwise known as rainout. When the humidifier is set in the system one mode, the ambient tracking is activated. The means that a patient will receive the same amount of moisture whether he or she is in the desert or by the ocean. When using the heated tubing, the temperature inside the tube is regulated allowing for consistent heat and moisture throughout the night. The home care company should be the ones in charge of changing the modes. The default mode is the system one with the ambient tracking activated. Of course, if a patient does not feel the need to use humidity, it can be turned off completely.

Pressing the button with the triangle activates the ramp. The home care company normally sets the length of time that the ramp is activated. You can request a specific time range dependent on how long you think it takes you to fall asleep. The range is from 5 minutes to 45 minutes.

The water chamber is dishwasher safe with the top and bottom separating from each other. The range for the Flex mode can be set from 1 to 3 to maximize breathing comfort.

The System One, 60 series, comes with a heated hose that can be used with the machine. It is inserted by simply lining up the ports on the hose with the port on the machine and pushing it in place. The entire System One series have automatic altitude adjustment for people that travel to different parts of the world. They also offer a Classic mode for the humidity and the System on mode. The classic mode only heat up the hot plate under the water chamber, and provides the moisture as the air flows through the chamber. The system one setting monitors the humidity level in the tube and auto regulates it to provide more consistent levels of humidity to the patient, thus reducing the condensation in the tube or the "rainout" that may cause the gurgling sound in the hose.

ResMed Tango

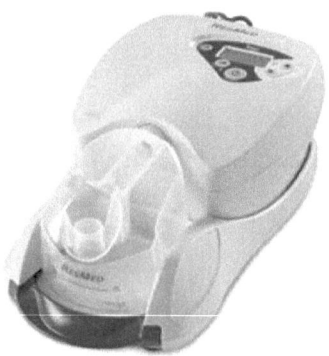

The Tango is the most basic of the CPAP models. It is solely a CPAP machine that offers straight pressure so you can breathe properly throughout the night. The range is from 4 to 20 cm H2O. It also comes equipped with a water chamber and it also has a ramp mode.

Fisher Paykel ICON

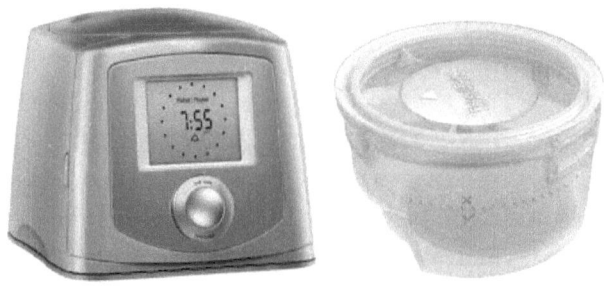

This machine offers an integrated clock and alarm with a chip that can be programed with up to 4 songs that can be used in lieu of the buzzer. This machine also offers the highest amount of humidity currently available on the market. It is good for patients who suffer from disorders like Sjogren's syndrome or are on strong diuretics.

The humidifier and CPAP are combined within the single unit and if requested, heated tubing can be added to the machine.   The heat setting in   the hose is set to   a constant temperature and is delivered by the copper coils in the hose. The hose is inserted into the back of the unit by simply lining it with the connection on the CPAP and pushing in till a slight click is felt. The Icon Auto offers Sensawake to maximize patient   comfort   while sleeping. It works inversely from the other pressure relief systems found on other machines.   The Sensawake is initiated when a patient starts arousing from sleep and the breathing pattern becomes more erratic.   Sensawake lowers the pressure till the patient falls back asleep and then increases the pressure back to therapeutic levels. This feature also allows the patient to remain asleep without out arousing during the night.   At   the   moment, the Sensawake feature is not offered in the CPAP mode. It also has automatic altitude compensation for those patients who travel often between sea level and the mountains.

To turn on the machine simply push in the middle silver button. You will hear a clicking sound and you will see the dots on the front of the screen travel around the screen. It takes a couple of seconds for the air to start flowing. The humidity can be adjusted by turning the outer silver ring one space from the 12 or top center position to the 1 o'clock position and pushing the center silver button. A thermometer will appear on the upper right side. You will also see a number on the front of the screen. To increase or decrease the number, push and hold the center button till the number starts blinking, then turn the outer ring to the right or left to increase or decrease the humidity level. Push the button again to stop the number from flashing and that will set the new humidity level. When the water chamber needs cleaning, it can be placed on the top rack of the dishwasher. As always, it is important to monitor the interior condition of the chamber to avoid the formation of mold on the bottom plate.

The ramp has a default setting of 20 minutes on the machine. To engage the ramp turn on the air and then push and hold the center button when the air is flowing till the ramp sign appears on the lower right side of the screen. It looks like a wedge. The starting pressure for this model is 4 cm of water pressure and also goes up to a pressure of 20.0 cm of water pressure.

DeVilbiss Intellipap CPAP

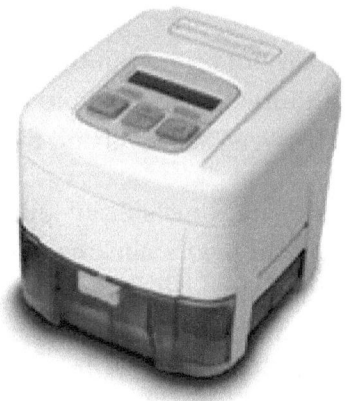

This machine can be bought with the optional integrated heated humidifier that sits under the CPAP. The Intellipap offers the Smart Flex technology that allows the pressure to lower with each exhalation, aiding in patient comfort. It also has an auto altitude adjustment up to 9000 feet, removing the worry of adequate pressure at higher altitudes.

This machine has the lowest CPAP setting on the market. The pressure on this machine can go as low as 3 cm of water pressure. It can be adjusted to a pressure of up to 20.0 cm of water pressure, just like all other CPAPs currently on the market. Because this CPAP is more compact than its competitors due to the water chamber sitting under the CPAP machine itself, it will occupy a smaller area on the nightstand.

CHAPTER TWELVE

Have CPAP, will Travel

To the universe and beyond!…with my CPAP

As many who start using CPAP have asked or wondered, what do I do if I need to travel? Most importantly, if you are accustomed to using your CPAP, never leave it at home. If you have read the first couple of chapters of this book, you are well aware how dangerous sleep apnea can be for the body and your health. So, leaving it for a couple of days or weeks will immediately put you at risk as you slide backwards towards that time when choking throughout the night was an constant occurrence.

The next thing to consider is how the machine will accompany you on your journey. If traveling on a plane, it is important to remember to not pack it in your luggage. Take the machine with you on the plane. The FAA recently ruled that people who travel by plane must be allowed to use devices like the CPAP on board. If your trip is not overnight, taking the CPAP with you will assure that you will have it available for use when you arrive at your destination. Just remember that CPAP's are considered life saving devices just like an oxygen tank. If you are traveling on a plane, a CPAP bag should never be considered a carry on. You can have as many carry-ons allowed by the airline PLUS your CPAP. If they start arguing with you, ask to speak to the supervisor. The exception for CPAP's is listed in their P&P manual. Another way around this potential dilemma is to always carry a letter of medical necessity from your doctor explaining your need for the machine.

It has not gotten easier to get the CPAP through the TSA security checkpoint, so it is important to try and make it as painless as possible. Remove the machine from its case and place it in its own bin. Since the bins are not clean, be prepared and store your CPAP in a plastic Ziplock before you leave your home, so you can remove it from its carrying case at the checkpoint and transfer it to the bin. Sometimes, the machine will have to undergo an Explosive Detection Test. This will occur after it is X-rayed. The officer will take the machine and run a small white swab over it and analyze the swab for any trace amounts of explosives. Please ask the person performing the test to first change their gloves, since the gloves are meant to protect them and not you or your machine. Once the check is completed, you will be able to store the machine back in its case and go merrily on your way. The best advice that can be given is to arrive at the airport earlier than normally recommended to allow extra time needed to get through the checkpoints without rushing and developing undue stress.

So, along with your carry-ons, the only other thing needed to make that CPAP machine work anywhere, is the plug that corresponds to electrical outlet in the country you are visiting. CPAP machines are also designed to automatically distinguish between 110 volts and 220 volts. All that is needed is the adapter plug to fit the American plug to the wall and an extension cord just in case the outlet is far away from the bed. With that taken care of, the machine should be ready for use. I am providing a link that will connect you to a site that lists all the outlets used throughout the world. It should make buying the correct plug easier.

http://www.kropla.com/electric2.htm

If you are an avid outdoors person, then traveling with your CPAP will present another set of problems; namely, how to run a CPAP without power. The answer is simple but somewhat complex all the same. The DC battery would be the obvious choice. Respironics, Puritan Bennett, ResMed have their own versions of battery packs that work their machines more esthetically pleasing. CPAP.com sells a lithium battery pack that weighs 2.5 lbs and can be recharged at any time without the risk of losing charge because of battery memory.

If that is not your biggest concern then head out the your local sporting goods store and ask for a DC battery that will run the machine for the night. Take into consideration that using the humidifier will require more energy, but normally if sleeping outdoors is part of the plan, then there should be enough humidity in the air to compensate for lack of a humidifier. If sleeping without a humidifier is not an option, there is a machine available on the market that may fit the bill rather well. It is the Transend CPAP with an integrated heat moisture exchange technology that uses the body's own moisture from each breath to maintain adequate humidity throughout the night.

Transcend Portable CPAP

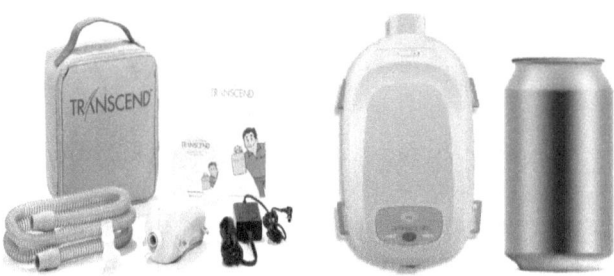

Currently the smallest CPAP on the market; weighing less than one pound with a cost of approximately $475.00, it fits in the palm of your hand. The Transcend CPAP offers the same pressure range as a traditional CPAP. It also eliminates the need for a humidifier by incorporating a disposable heat moisture exchange piece that uses the body's own moisture to maintain the necessary humidification. It can be worn attached to the top of the head or resting above the pillow. It includes a ramp mode from 5 to 45 minutes. It does not have the Flexing or pressure relief feature that most other machines on the market provide, but if a patient is using it for travel and he or she can manage sleeping without that feature, this CPAP fills a much needed niche. The pressure will automatically adjust so that it maintains the correct pressure prescribed for the patient up to an altitude of 8000 ft., so there is no need to have the pressure changed before traveling to higher or lower altitudes. . If humidity is a major concern than consider buying a machine that has an integrated humidifier since the moisture exchange system on the Transcend, may leave some patients with a greater need for that moisture somewhat lacking.

The website also offers several portable batteries that

can be used for any make of CPAP. They are light weigh and will last throughout the night.

Another site that is worth perusing is the following.

http://www.thebatterygeeks.com

This site sells batteries and also rents to own batteries for use with your CPAP. The rent to own option allows you to buy and pay for a battery over a three-month period. In this manner, the burden of payment is lessened, especially since the batteries needed for camping, boating, or RVing are not covered by insurance.

CHAPTER THIRTEEN

Avoiding the Doctor "Void"

Diagnosis is not the end, but the beginning of practice

Martin H. Fischer

In all the years that I have worked in this field, I have noticed that one of the biggest problems that many patients face is the gap between the initial consult, the sleep studies, the report of the results of the studies, and the next step. What brought this to my attention was a phone call that I received from a patient asking for his results. One of the administrative assistants in the lab went to get his file and when she brought it to me we both looked at it and realized that this poor patient had had a sleep study two years earlier and swore that he had never been contacted by anyone with the outcome. Hard to believe, you may say. I thought so...but there was no notation from a doctor or any other health professional in his chart stating otherwise.

We called the referring doctor's office and asked if the patient had been followed up on their end and received the response that they had assumed that we taken over his care. The patient, trusting in the "efficiency" of the medical profession, waited for a call or letter that never came. The patient suffered needlessly because each office assumed that the other was in charge of following up with the patient. The other failsafe that broke down was with the patient itself. He never called with the relevant questions.

This black hole is ever-present in the medical profession. With so many specialists being seen by so many patients, the stream of information can be hindered or halted by a lack of communication. How can a patient remedy this? Simply take charge of your health!

Keep copies of all reports by all physicians in a file at home. Bring the relevant information to visits with new doctors to help to them better understand your complaints or conditions. Never assume that all doctors offices are in contact with each other. Most are not unless they exist within a network that has a central information network where the different practices are connected. Even with that connection in place, you cannot completely compensate for the human element that can "drop the ball". The medical field is being overwhelmed with a flood of new patients daily. The baby boomers, the largest generation to reach old age, are assailing the medical field with varied conditions brought on in part, by age, general lifestyle, and overall attitude. Doctors, nurses, technicians, technologists and all other staff are being stretched to the limit so imperative that we, as patients, help to lighten the load by being proactive in our health.

The Internet also can confound medical care. The saying, "A little knowledge is a dangerous thing" is especially relevant in this instance. I have had to deal with many patients who walk in to my lab filled with tidbits of information that confuse them and which can, at times, increase levels of anxiety. The Internet, though an amazing tool, is a place fraught with misleading information, false leads, and gimmicks. It is important for the patient to take whatever information acquired through the Internet with a grain of salt until the information has been verified by trusted sources.

Case in point...the oral appliance. There are ads scattered throughout the internet touting the benefits of oral appliances similar to mouth guards that almost guarantee that anyone using them will surely stop having sleep apnea and never snore again. The cost of the "wonder " mouth inserts is small compared to the amount that a patient would pay to have one made at a Sleep certified dentist. I admit that the initial cost is extremely tempting and there **may** be some relief from snoring, but bear in mind that these gadgets are one size fits all. I don't recall anyone having a mouth that is exactly like someone else's...except for identical twins; and I doubt that they are truly identical. So just keep in mind that cheaper may not be better and always analyze the data with a critical eye, especially when it comes to sleeping.

I once had a patient who came to see me who was completely frustrated with his care. He had certain co-morbidities that had baffled most of the doctors that he had seen. He went on to tell me that the final straw occurred when one of the doctors he was seeing proceeded to tell him that he was going to search the Internet for a solution. The patient was thunderstruck. He told me that he could have been equally as capable of searching the internet but he had decided to go to a doctor for medical expertise; so why was he paying this doctor an enormous amount for an office visit when he was going to do the same thing the patient could do from the comfort of his own house. I responded that being a doctor allowed him access to sites not normally open to the layperson where he could search for information through journal articles based on research studies. He could also consult with colleagues online to search for possible answers. He was somewhat mollified by my answers, though not entirely. As is evident in the above example; the way doctors talk to patients is critical. Too little information and the patient feels cheated; too much, and the patient can become confused, anxious, or downright belligerent.

If the proper balance can be found between patient and physician and the proper line of communication can be established, then proper care should be able to be delivered to the satisfaction of both parties. If you have a doctor who ignores your requests, find another doctor. As in everything, there are good doctors and bad ones. You, as the patient, must also realize that medicine is not an exact science. It is through curiosity, research, luck, and at times, plain old detective work, that answers can be found to confounding questions. Not all doctors will have the answers, which is why the second opinion is so important. BE PROACTIVE about your health and you will lead a better life.

CHAPTER FOURTEEN

Muddling through the Internet wasteland

*Getting information off the Internet is like taking a
drink from a fire hydrant*

Mitch Kapor, variation of a quote by Jerome Weisner

So now that the CPAP has become yours, all these other factors come into play. If you have read this book to this point, most of your questions should have been answered. Unfortunately, medicine is an ever-changing field and as such, new information, cures, adaptations or concepts will always be present. It is because of this that I am listing the most relevant internet sites that may help those interested to search more efficiently for answers to questions that may not have been answered. These will include:

1: major corporate sites

2: sources for products...especially if insurance or the lack of it is an issue

3: chat sites for those who want to vent or inform others about their CPAP experience

4: sites set up as charity for those who desperately need a CPAP but cannot afford a new one.

The Big four Companies that make CPAP are, in no particular order, ResMed, Respironics, Fisher Paykel and

Devilbiss. Their sites are descriptive, nice to look at and fairly user friendly. If you are not the average computer geek, then some sites may be a little more challenging to surf than others. The sites are a good starting point to look at the newest products on the market for CPAP users. They are informative and offer a more in-depth analysis of their products. Another source for information is offered by the NIH(National Institute of Health) the website is called Medlineplus:

www.nlm.nih.gov/medlineplus

The site offers information about CPAP, homeopathic medicines available on the market for anxiety, insomnia and natural aids that help in calming the body so a person can fall asleep. It is an objective, informative site that will aid the reader in making informed decisions about how to manage their health.

Merchandise cannot be bought on any of these sites, so if you are looking to buy, please contact your DME provider or one of the online sites that sell CPAP supplies.

If your are looking to buy online then the biggest sites for CPAP supplies and the most reputable that I have encountered are:

www.cpapwholesale.com
www.CPAP.com
www.cpapman.com
www.1800cpap.com

These sites have been in business for years. Please remember that these sites are great for people with limited insurance coverage. The prices are competitive but you must remember that the warranties offered are only those of the manufacturers. The individual websites do not service customers like local home care companies.

CPAP machines bought online are significantly cheaper than if the same machine is purchased from the DME provider. The biggest difference is that many providers will work with you if something goes wrong with the CPAP by replacing the units with rentals till the problem can be resolved. They will then contact the manufacturers and get the units fixed or replaced, taking the burden off of the customer. If you buy your CPAP online and something breaks, you are only covered by the 2–3 year warranty and you have to contact the manufacturer directly. It can become a hassle, but if this is the only option, then it is the best way to go.

When it comes to finding out information about certain aspects of CPAP that are not readily available, then the discussion boards may be of help. Below are listed a couple of good websites,

www.apneaboard.com

www.cpaptalk.com

Most of the chatter comes from fellow CPAP users. Remember that what is posted is the opinion of the individual respondent and some of the responses may not be useful. It can also be quite confusing since the responses to certain questions can vary greatly, at times. All in all, the sites can offer a different perspective to the whole CPAP experience. I have read stories posted by different people, seen comic strips made up about CPAP, read jokes and have gotten insight into the feelings and at times, bias associated with using a CPAP.

You can find and make friends who will support you and help you on your journey. You will find a shoulder to cry on, a rock to stand on, and the breath of thousands of people who use CPAP nightly that will fill your sheets and coax you forward as you breathe each breath with your life saving device. So peruse these sites and join a couple of them; adding your voice and your opinions to the groups. You never know...your input may help another who is floundering as you once may have done yourself.

If, hopefully, you reach that point where CPAP has become a part of your life a funny thing may start to happen over time... the supplies sent to you by your DME provider will start piling up. Not knowing what to do with them, the majority are saved, stockpiled away in a drawer or closet; mostly out of guilt about throwing away brand new supplies. Since this is a concern for many who presently have unused accessories, donating them is a feasible solution. In this manner, your stockpile is reduced significantly and you help those who are less fortunate.

One thing that I should mention...DME companies should not normally send you supplies without your consent. Previously, this was something that occurred frequently, but insurance companies ar cracking down with this type of excess, so ask your provider if you can call instead when you need supplies. In this manner, you will only receive what you need.

Over the years, I have had patients ask me if there was

any way that their older CPAP's could be recycled or donated. Initially, that was not an option, but as the use of CPAP becomes more prevalent, more and more machines are being socked away in closets, garages, bedrooms, etc as patients upgrade to newer models. For those of you fortuitous enough to have been "upgraded" and nice enough to care about helping others here are some sites that currently are accepting gently used CPAP machines:

http://www.reggiewhitefoundation.

http://www.herofargo.org
(Project Hero-Healthcare Equipment Recycling Organization)

http://sleepapnea.org
(The American Sleep Apnea association)

http://www.secondwindcpap.com

Also contact local hospitals, DME providers, and the Visiting Nurses Association in your area to find out if they recycle or can put you in contact with an organization that provides used CPAPs to those less fortunate. The local church or synagogue may also offer another alternative to help other members of the community receive much needed equipment.

http://www.youneedsleep.com

This is another company that allows you to donate your CPAP to help those in need. They also offer discounted machines and masks for people who do not have an insurance plan that adequately covers the needs of the patient.

When you finally find an individual or an agency that accepts machines, please keep in mind that the condition of the unit is very important. The machines and accessories that will be donated must be in gently used condition. **CPAP's from smokers, or that have been abused, that are ten   years old or older, will not be accepted.** They must be in good working order and preferably with low usage hours. They should also come with the original manuals that were included in the package. Make sure that you clean the machine, put in a new filter and clean the water chamber.

CHAPTER FIFTEEN

Everything in a nutshell- a quick reference to everything CPAP

Efficiency is doing things right; effectiveness is doing the right things

Peter Drucker

In a nutshell, you have to be efficient and effective when dealing with CPAP. The efficiency comes into play when maintaining the machine and the accessories related to the machine; namely, hoses, masks, filters, water chambers and the exterior of the machine itself. The effectiveness is related to how often the machine is used.

CPAP is not something that can be used sporadically. If it is not used on a regular basis, the body starts to drift down that slide of negative feedback. CPAP is not a cure. It is a tool that is needed by those who have sleep apnea, to maintain a good quality of life. It does not cure sleep apnea, it just prevents it from happening through the use of pressurized air. Remember that gravity, our friend in the daytime, is the constant that undermines our sleep at night. It presses down on our throats and forces its collapse when the opportunity arises. So in a nutshell, here are points that should be addressed when CPAP is used.

1. There is a learning curve.

For many of you just starting the journey, using CPAP will be tough. If you notice that you take the mask off at night, do not fret, put it on again the next night and try to sleep. Give your body time to adjust, for the majority of you, it will.

2. Do not be afraid to ask for help.

If this book was not sufficient, then please call the lab or the DME provider who set you up, if you don't know how to use your equipment or how to put on a mask. They have trained staff that should be able to address your concerns and help you to get comfortable with your machine.

3. Maintain your equipment.

Clean and wipe down masks, hoses, machines and change filters frequently and wash out your water chamber at least once per week

4. Replace your accessories often.

Filters should be changed or washed once every three months, The black filters that look like sponges can be washed and reused. Most of the white filters are disposable and need to be replaced. If you have pets then once a month...mask every six months, hoses once per year.

5. Don't suffer with "bad" mask.

Again, your DME or Home care provider should be able to help you get fitted with a mask that "fits" you. There are constant advances being made in sleep related equipment so don't throw in the proverbial towel, keep trying to find the right fit. For some, just one mask fits perfectly; for others, alternating between different masks works best.

6. Don't be conned by false promises.

I have to comment on the vast amount of sites that promise suffers of sleep apnea that "miracle" cure. Some sites offer herbal remedies, other sites offer new fangled gizmos claiming to that hold the airway open as you sleep. Please remember that there is nothing that can really be done to stop the force of gravity bearing down on you. It just does so relentlessly and there are no magic pills that can be taken to prevent that. Diet and exercise may help you to lose weight and thus reduce the size of your neck, but that does not mean that you can come off of your machine. The only way to know for sure is through a sleep study. If you are diagnosed with a mild case of sleep apnea, there are other forms of treatment that may resolve the problem. Talk to a board certified sleep doctor that can lead you in the right directions.

7. You can't suffocate when using CPAP.

I often get asked the question...What happens if the lights go off or I lose power. That actually happened one night when I working in a lab in Florida, the lightening capital of the world. I was a newbie in the field of sleep medicine and I panicked, to say the least. I grabbed a flashlight and ran into the patients' rooms to take off the mask to let them breathe. When I went into the first room, I saw the patient on CPAP started having the classic apneas that they had lived with for years. Before I could take off the mask, patient woke up and ripped it off. He sat up in the bed slightly disoriented. I calmed him down and rushed to the other patient. Amazingly, other patient was still asleep! I could see how his body was struggling to suck in air through the small open port. As I went to take off the mask, the power came on. In total, it was off only for a couple of minutes...two to three at most. I was able quickly turn the machine back on and the patient continued sleeping, none the wiser. I was surprised that he slept through the power outage, but as I later learned, when a patient is extremely sleep deprived the brain will try to maintain a state of sleep for as long as possible. Since this person had not slept well for years, it would have taken longer for him to arouse and rip off the mask; but rest assured that it would have happened sooner rather than later. How do I know this?

Because over the years, patients have recounted an innumerable times how they had unknowingly taken off their masks due to discomfort or lack of air. In short, the brain will not allow you NOT to breathe. It will rip the mask off if it is not getting the needed air, especially if you have been on CPAP for a while. Also, there are safety valves on the masks that open when the pressure is turned off. This will allow air into the mask. Not enough for you to breathe comfortably, but enough to not suffocate. Either way, the patient will always survive a short-term power outage. If you are still fretting over the remote possibility, then invest in a surge protector with a battery backup that lasts one hour or a generator and fall asleep without worries.

8. "Break" the seal.

When trying to separate the mask from the hose break the seal by placing one hand on the connector of the mask at the base and another on the rubber portion of the hose. Bend both as if you were trying to bend steel...just imagine you are Superman. This will allow air to enter, breaking the seal holding one to the other. Remember that the hose is designed to withstand the tossing and turning in bed, which pulls on whatever is attached to you including your mask and hose. The end of the hose is tacky for that specific reason. I have seen an innumerable number of patients with parts missing from their masks because they pulled on the hose and mask to separate them only to unknowingly leave a part of the mask stuck to the hose. I even got a desperate call from a patient because the mask that had been shipped out to him by his home care company was not fitting on his hose. After an extended conversation with both the patient and his wife, I realized that the plastic fitting that belonged to the previous mask, was still attached to the hose. Once it was removed, the new mask fit perfectly. They were amazed that such a minor issue could cause such grief. Just remember, if you hold on to the hose and the mask on both ends and break them apart as if you were breaking a loaf of bread, or as if you were bending a steel rod; the seal will be broken and the hose will separate easily.

9. Have CPAP ...will travel

CPAP machines are made to automatically distinguish between 110 volts and 220 volts. All that is needed is the adapter plug to fit the American plug to the wall. A CPAP is considered to be a life-saving device just like an oxygen tank. In plane travel, a CPAP bag should never be considered a carry on. Take it with you. Do not pack it into your suitcase, BUT you can have as many carry-ons allowed by the airline PLUS your CPAP. If they start arguing with you, ask to speak to the supervisor. The exception for CPAP's is listed in their P&P manual. And is backed by the Americans with disabilities act. If you are an avid camper, there are DC batteries available that work with several CPAP models. Respironics, Puritan Bennett, ResMed have their own versions of battery packs. CPAP.com sells a lithium battery pack that weighs 2.5 lbs and can be recharged at any time without the risk of losing charge because of battery memory. When camping, you should not use the humidifier. Using a humidifier will run down the battery faster and because you are outdoors, you really should have no need for the humidification. Lithium batteries are also made that support CPAP.

CHAPTER SIXTEEN

What if you hate CPAP...Other alternatives and Holistic avenues for better sleep

Nothing is so good that somebody, somewhere will not hate it.

Pohl's Law

Often, I come across patients who simply cannot adapt to using CPAP. The majority of these patients fall in the mild range when they are diagnosed. With many of these patients, the sleep apnea can either be positional (when it occurs mainly while sleeping on their back), or REM related. In these instances, the brain fights back, in a sense. It will accept CPAP when it is needed, but will reject the forced air when no events are occurring. For patients who suffer this type of scenario, the only alternative that may exist is the discontinuation of CPAP and the commencement of alternative treatment modalities. One of the newest of these is the Provent sleep apnea therapy.

Provent is an FDA approved therapy that consists of one way valves that are affixed to the front of the nostrils, covering the nasal passageways. The Provent tabs are held in place by an adhesive that secures the device to the nose. The Air flows freely into the body when inhalation occurs but when breathing out, a back flow or resistance occurs during exhalation. This backpressure is equivalent to a CPAP pressure of approximately 8.0 cm

H2O to 10.0 cm H2O; though, currently there is no way to measure that while the patient is using the tabs. It helps to hold the airway open as the breathing transitions from breathing out to breathing in. Many state that it felt somewhat uncomfortable when initially starting up with Provent, but after a couple of days to about one week, the initial sensation of discomfort dissipated. Provent allows patients with mild to moderate sleep apnea to breathe better at night without using a CPAP. It can be a good alternative for patients who do a lot of traveling since it can be utilized nightly without the cumbersome accessories that come along with using a CPAP. Their site states that for many who have tried Provent, their snoring has decreased about 60% while on the device. The biggest downside to Provent is that it currently is not covered by insurance. The cost of buying a month's worth is approximately $60 – $85 dollars.

The oral appliance or mandibular advancement device (M.A.D.) is another option that has been studied and has proven to be a fairly good alternative for patients with mild to moderate OSA. The name describes precisely what the device does. It is meant to jut the lower jaw forward. When you jut your lower jaw so that the lower teeth are in front of the upper teeth, you are hyperextending the jaw. But it is that ability that allows people who cannot tolerate a CPAP to have success with this device. The greater the range of movement forward, the more the airway in the back of the throat opens up. Normally a clinic visit with your sleep doctor is needed to ascertain if you are a candidate. Things that are considered are the shape and range of movement of the jaw. Other factors include whether or not a patient has suffered from TMJ (temporal mandibular joint) syndrome, which is signaled by a clicking noise in the jaw when it moves up and down or sideways. Using an oral appliance would only exacerbate the problem causing further discomfort. Patients who have had implants in the mouth also have to be excluded as possible candidates. But if all is in order you will be referred to a board certified sleep dentist who specializes in these types of devices. The device fits inside the mouth and covers both the upper and lower teeth. There is a screw that can protrude from the front of the device, or a hinge that connects the two pieces together. These mechanisms are what are used to move the lower jaw, or mandible forward. The more the mechanism is adjusted, the greater the displacement of the jaw. This then opens the back of the throat and adds tension to the throat, reducing snoring and allowing for less restriction and greater airflow.

A good place to start looking for a board Certified Sleep Dentist is the Academy of Dental Sleep Medicine,

(www. dentalsleepmed.org).

Their site offers a list of dentists who are experienced in measuring and fitting patients with the device. The appliance may be covered by insurance if the doctor can present a good case to the insurance company, but in the majority of instances, neither the medical insurance nor the dental insurance will cover the cost of the device. The out of pocket cost can range from approximately $700.00 to $1500.00 dollars. One other thing to keep in mind is that the devices can break or wear out, incurring additional costs for replacement.

The Didgeridoo. An aboriginal instrument that if used consistently over the long term, helps to strengthen the throat muscles precisely where snoring and apneas occur.. It is theorized that it is the combination of the low vibratory tone made by the instrument and the learned technique of circular breathing that helps to reduce snoring and decrease the incidence of events in patients who have mild to moderate sleep apnea.

In order to be able to play the didgeridoo a technique called circular breathing has to be learned. There are several videos that can be found on U-Tube that demonstrate how to learn this process. One of the better ones is a series of videos by Ondrej Smeykal titled:

Ondrej Smeykal - How to Circular Breathe

He explains in detail the steps necessary to properly learn the technique. If this is something that peeks your interest didgeridoos can be bought for as little as thirty dollars, with the price increasing depending on the quality of the instrument. Suffice to say that for the purpose of reducing snoring or sleep apnea, a cheap one would suffice. You can also search Youtube.com and the internet in general for instructions on building your own.

Snoring U is an Apple app that helps monitor a person's snoring while sleeping. The app is downloaded onto a smartphone and when turned on, the phone is placed under the pillow. It app supposedly registers the degree of snoring and vibrates or "nudges" the person causing a slight arousal and hopefully, shift, helping then to stop the snoring. The app records the snoring and amplitude throughout the entire night and marks when the snoring was loudest on a graph. It also shows the number of times the "nudge feature" was implemented throughout the night. The data can then be downloaded onto a computer or laptop and a record of the intensity and amount of snoring throughout the night can be seen through the colored graphs that are displayed on the screen. The app also records the snoring so the person can actually listen to their snoring during the night. In short, the app allows a person to become more aware of their snoring and maybe motivate him or her to take action to help remedy the problem.

Rematee ...(www...rematee.com) is a fairly new product that is being used for positional therapy. Sometimes patients who are diagnosed with mild to moderate sleep apnea have the events only when they are on their back. When the patient shifts to the side, the events stop. That is where an aid like Rematee could be very useful. It is a holter made from Neoprene with two straps that rest over the shoulders and are attached to the "belt" that fits around the upper body or torso. On the back there are four pockets where inflatable plastic cylinders can be inserted. When all the pockets are in use and the cylinders are fully inflated, they prevent the patient from rolling onto their back. As far as shifting from side to side, the patient would them have to learn to turn on to their stomach first, in order to shift to the other side.

The Rematee is also sold with a tee shirt that is made from all natural materials and along with the halter, is machine washable. The Rematee comes in different sizes with a starting cost of about 150.00 dollars. It is only sold online at the moment, but the website offers a 1-800 number to call with any questions. Presently, it is not covered by insurance.

Last, there are several holistic aids that may aid in helping people to relax and allow them to fall asleep more quickly. Besides using warm milk or a hot bath to soothe the muscles and calm the mind, consider trying the following. (As a note, please investigate thoroughly any holistic supplements before diving in and trying them. Some of them can interact negatively with current medications that you may be taking so be forewarned and go forth with care.)

Valarian root - Known to have sedating properties though there is not enough clinical evidence that it consistently works well. As with many holistic treatments, success varies from patient to patient.

L-theanine in combination with fish oil - Also is used for anxiety because of its calming effects on the body. L-theanine is an amino acid that is derived from green tea leaves. It has been used in Japan for decades with no side effects ever noted. I have had patients tell me that since they have started taking the products, many "sleep like babies". Other patients have noticed that their sleep is deeper, and their awakenings are less frequent during the night.

Vitamin B12 - Taking this vitamin at night helps many patients sleep better at night because it influences the production of melatonin in the body. It causes the melatonin to be released into the system earlier thus promoting sleep. People who have taken it have reported to sleep more deeply. Since it is a water-soluble vitamin, if taken in excess, the extra vitamin B12 will be flushed out through urination.

Melatonin - An amino acid that is naturally produced in the body and is the key component to promote sleep. The supplements that are sold on the market aid those who have difficulty with sleep onset. It must be taken at the beginning of the night for greatest effect. Then it works in conjunction with the melatonin produced in the body and helps the body to fall asleep naturally. If a person wakes up later and takes melatonin, there is no effect. This could be due, in part to how the sleep cycle works in the body.

Exercise - It does two things. First, it produces endorphins in the body that are considered mood elevators. Second, it just plain tires you out! If done at least three hours before bedtime, it should help the body to relax and prepare for bed more readily since the body is more inclined to sleep to help repair the muscles and detoxify the body after a good workout. Over time, exercising will allow the body to go into a deeper stage of sleep and it will help you to wake up more refreshed.

Using CPAP is an adventure. For many, the road will be long and arduous; for others, it will be like a leisurely stroll through the park. Whatever your path, just remember...with good habits before going to sleep, a positive frame of mind and most importantly...perseverance, the hurdles will be overcome and the ultimate war against poor sleep will be won.

Good luck and good night to you all!

REFERENCES

1: Selim B, Won C, Yaggi HK. Cardiovascular consequences of sleep apnea. Clin Chest Med. 2010 Jun;31(2):203-20. Review. PubMed PMID: 20488282.

2: Yaggi HK, Strohl KP. Adult obstructive sleep apnea/hypopnea syndrome: definitions, risk factors, and pathogenesis. Clin Chest Med. 2010 Jun;31(2):179-86. Review. PubMed PMID: 20488280.

3: Kapur VK, Baldwin CM, Resnick HE, Gottlieb DJ, Nieto FJ. Sleepiness in patients with moderate to severe sleep-disordered breathing. Sleep. 2005 Apr;28(4):472-7. PubMed PMID: 16171292.

4: Urbano F, Roux F, Schindler J, Mohsenin V. Impaired cerebral autoregulation in obstructive sleep apnea. J Appl Physiol. 2008 Dec;105(6):1852-7. Epub 2008 Oct16. PubMed PMID: 18927265.

5: D'Ambrosio C, Bowman T, Mohsenin V. Quality of life in patients with obstructive sleep apnea: effect of nasal continuous positive airway pressure—a prospective study.

6: Otake K, Delaive K, Walld R, Manfreda J, Kryger MH. Cardiovascular medication use in patients with undiagnosed obstructive sleep apnoea. Thorax. 2002 May;57(5):417-22. PubMed PMID: 11978918; PubMed Central PMCID: PMC1746332.

7: Selim B, Won C, Yaggi HK. Cardiovascular consequences of sleep apnea. Clin Chest Med. 2010 Jun;31(2):203-20. Review. PubMed PMID: 20488282.

8: Heinzer RC, Pellaton C, Rey V, Rossetti AO, Lecciso G, Haba-Rubio J, Tafti M, Lavigne G. Positional therapy for obstructive sleep apnea: An objective measurement of patients' usage and efficacy at home. Sleep Med. 2012 Apr;13(4):425-8. Epub 2012 Jan 18. PubMed PMID: 22261242.

9: Filtness AJ, Reyner LA, Horne JA. One night's CPAP withdrawal in otherwise compliant OSA patients: marked driving impairment but good awareness of increased sleepiness. Sleep Breath. 2011 Sep 6. [Epub ahead of print] PubMed PMID:21898097.

10: Mason RH, Kiire CA, Groves DC, Lipinski HJ, Jaycock A, Winter BC, Smith L,Bolton A, Rahman NM, Swaminathan R, Chong VN, Stradling JR. Visual
Improvement following Continuous Positive Airway Pressure Therapy in Diabetic Subjects with Clinically Significant Macular Oedema and Obstructive Sleep Apnoea: Proof of Principle Study. Respiration. 2011 Dec 20. [Epub ahead of print] PubMed PMID: 22189259.

11: Filtness AJ, Reyner LA, Horne JA. One night's CPAP withdrawal in otherwise compliant OSA patients: marked driving impairment but good awareness of increased sleepiness. Sleep Breath. 2011 Sep 6. [Epub ahead of print] PubMed PMID:21898097.12: Kushida CA, Berry RB, Blau A, Crabtree T, Fietze I, Kryger MH, Kuna ST, Pegram GV Jr, Penzel T. Positive airway pressure initiation: a randomized controlled trial to assess the impact of therapy mode and titration process on efficacy,adherence, and outcomes. Sleep. 2011 Aug 1;34(8):1083-92. PubMed PMID: 21804670; PubMed Central PMCID: PMC3138163.

13: Valentin A, Subramanian S, Quan SF, Berry RB, Parthasarathy S. Air leak is associated with poor adherence to autoPAP therapy. Sleep.2011 Jun 1;34(6):801-6. PubMed PMID: 21629369; PubMed Central PMCID: PMC3098948.

14: Walsh JK, Griffin KS, Forst EH, Ahmed HH, Eisenstein RD, Curry DT, Hall-Porter JM, Schweitzer PK. A convenient expiratory positive airway pressure nasal device for the treatment of sleep apnea in patients non-adherent with continuous positive airway pressure. Sleep Med. 2011 Feb;12(2):147-52. Epub 2011 Jan 21.PubMed PMID: 21256800.

15: Buchner NJ, Quack I, Stegbauer J, Woznowski M, Kaufmann A, Rump LC. Treatment of obstructive sleep apnea reduces arterial stiffness. Sleep Breath. 2012 Mar;16(1):123-33. Epub 2011 Jan 7. PubMed PMID: 21213062.

16: Bianchi MT, Eiseman NA, Cash SS, Mietus J, Peng CK, Thomas RJ. Probabilistic sleep architecture models in patients with and without sleep apnea. J Sleep Res. 2011 Sep 28. doi: 10.1111/j.1365-2869.2011.00937.x. [Epub ahead of print] PubMed PMID: 21955148.

17: Djonlagic I, Saboisky J, Carusona A, Stickgold R, Malhotra A. Increased sleep fragmentation leads to impaired off-line consolidation of motor memories in humans. PLoS One. 2012;7(3):e34106. Epub 2012 Mar 28. PubMed PMID: 22470524.

18: Shah NA, Yaggi HK, Concato J, Mohsenin V. Obstructive sleep apnea as a risk factor for coronary events or cardiovascular death. Sleep Breath. 2010 Jun;14(2):131-6. Epub 2009 Sep 24. PubMed PMID: 19777281.

19: Stephen R. Thompson, Uwe Ackermann, Richard L. Horner. Sleep as a teaching tool for integrating respiratory physiology and motor control. Advances in Physiology Education. March 2012, 36 (1). Print ISSN: 1043-4046, Online ISSN:1522-1229

About the author

A graduate of the University of Connecticut, Elizabeth Lowe has been in the field of sleep technology for over a decade. She earned her RPSGT from the Board of Sleep Technologists and is a Registered Sleep tech with the American Board of Sleep Medicine. Elizabeth has worked as the lead day tech at Yale University in the department of Sleep Medicine helping patients become acclimated to using CPAP and aiding patients in incorporating CPAP into their daily routines with great success for over seven years. She also continues to work nights at Hartford Hospital running sleep studies and providing CPAP therapy to patients who qualify. She currently resides in Connecticut.

www.ingramcontent.com/pod-product-compliance
Lightning Source LLC
Chambersburg PA
CBHW030446290526
45786CB00001B/466